Ce
Elimi   *st*

Natural Therapies for Effective Cellulite Treatments

By Marta Tuchowska

New Revised Edition - November 2015

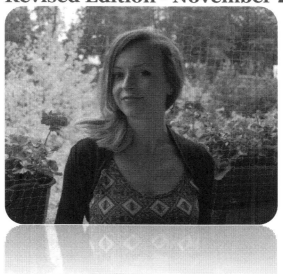

www.holisticwellnessproject.com
www.amazon.com/author/mtuchowska

All information in this book has been carefully researched and checked for factual accuracy. However, the author and publishers make no warranty, expressed or implied, that the information contained herein is appropriate for every individual, situation or purpose, and assume no responsibility for errors or omission. The reader assumes the risk and full responsibility for all actions, and the author will not be held liable for any loss or damage, whether consequential, incidental, and special or otherwise, that may result from the information presented in this publication.

A physician has not written the information in this book. Before making any serious dietary changes, I advise you to consult with your physician first.

<u>Introduction</u> Cellulite Killers...7

If you are thinking: "Does it really work?", it's time to change your mindset. It DOES work! Cellulite Killers are a secret alliance of Natural Therapies that do not aim at eliminating cellulite alone. They do their best and always manage to kill the <u>causes of cellulite</u> so that you can relax and go shopping for your dream bikini now! Eradicating the causes makes more sense than only eradicating the effect, right?

<u>Chapter 1:</u>Holistic Therapies and Cellulite...22

In this chapter I will try to change your mindset about cellulite and teach you how to perceive everything, especially cellulite, in a holistic way. I will also share my personal story and hopefully give you a realistic view to prepare your own action plan using the methods that helped me. Holistic health before cellulite is just like wellness before Weight Loss. True beauty comes from health.

<u>Chapter2:</u>Your Friends and Your Enemies...24

It's time to analyze your lifestyle and get to the root of the problem. Be your own coach, you can do it! In order to fight cellulite, we must first realize our weapons and recognize our enemies also. If you believe in mind over matter, don't skip this chapter. It will help you prepare an accurate action plan for your cellulite battle.

<u>Chapter3:</u>Caffeine and Cellulite...32

In this day and age, most people crawl out of bed and the first thing they do is to drink a cup of coffee. There are more coffee addicts than we actually think. How does coffee influence our cellulite problem? Is coffee and caffeine our friend or our enemy? Actually- both, depending on how you use them! You will also learn to substitute coffee with other, more nutritious drinks. Trust me, it does matter in the cellulite battle.

Chapter4:Phytotherapy and Herbs...40

This is going to be our first proper treatment 'from the inside'. In this chapter I share a very specific phytotherapy recipe that is really effective for treating cellulite. You will also learn all about each herb from the blend as well as how to use them separately.

Additionally, you will learn other therapeutic indications of the herbs mentioned and you will be able to apply them to alleviate other common-ailments that you, or your loved-ones, might be suffering from.

Chapter5:Aromatherapy and Spa Treatments...48

In this chapter I will show you some additional, yet also very effective anti-cellulite treatments that you can create with aromatherapy. If you are a spa lover, this chapter will teach you how to pamper yourself by creating your own, inexpensive mini spa. You will also learn the basic rules of aromatherapy for holistic spa treatments, not only for cellulite but also for other common ailments

Chapter6:Balanced Nutrition (not just an Anti-Cellulite *Diet!*)...48

This chapter will inspire you towards healthy and balanced nutrition so as to correct certain imbalances that may be causing your cellulite condition or contributing to it. Use my listings as a reference and feel free to adapt it to your lifestyle, taste bud preferences and of course, your health goals.

Chapter7:Exercise...59

They say: 'no pain no gain'. I say: 'no pleasure no gain' because exercise can also be fun. It all comes down to your attitude that may need to be shifted towards a healthily active lifestyle.

This chapter will put you right back on track. Brush yourself off and jump back on the wagon if you really want to KILL that cellulite and show off that sexy bikini!

Chapter8:Lymphatic Massage...62

I am a certified massage therapist and lymphatic drainage massage has always been my favorite treatment. In this chapter I will explain to you all the benefits that regular lymphatic drainage massage brings. It is a great additional treatment to detoxify your body and give some real pleasure to your senses...

Chapter9:BONUS: Eliminating Cellulite with the Alkaline Diet...65

Learn which foods are alkalizing and restore balance. Reduce cellulite with alkaline foods and get your energy back. All you need to understand about alkalinity and additional recipes to get started. Re-balancing your pH means less cellulite. It's really simple.

Chapter10:BONUS: Eliminate Cellulite with Yoga, Pilates and Physical Activity...71

All you need to know about yoga, pilates and more effective workouts that you can do wherever you want and whenever you want. Make fitness and relaxation your lifestyle.

Conclusion: Winning the Battle...91

My final thoughts to keep you motivated during the cellulite final battle process. Keep on the famous TRACK of health. Be good on yourself, don't try to be perfect but aim for progress. Learn how to trick your brain to take action, even when you have a bad day or don't feel motivated.

JOIN MY FREE HOLISTIC WELLNESS NEWSLETTER

Join my wellness + holistic lifestyle design newsletter and get free instant access to my guide: "Revolutionize Your Life with Alkaline Foods" + my insider news, amazing
free bonuses + plenty of healthy recipes + receive all my upcoming books for free or 99c.

Start creating a happy body, mind and spirit today! Subscribe here: www.bitly.com/AlkalineMarta
Or here: www.holisticwellnessproject.com/alkaline-diet-ebook/giveaway.html

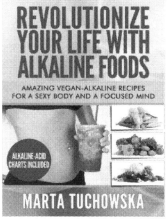

No SPAM. I hate SPAM as much as you do. The reason why I have a mailing list is to connect with my readers and help them create wellness and health. Let's keep in touch!

Introduction

Dear Reader, thank you for purchasing the book: *Cellulite Killers: Eliminate Cellulite Fast*. Let me tell you that contrary to its title, this is not just another guide addressed only to those suffering from cellulite. Everyone can read and benefit from it, even those lucky ones who have never been struck by cellulite attacks (I do envy them!).

The treatments I mention in this book will also help you gain more energy and improve your overall health. Irrespective of your age, sex or occupation, you can apply the treatments from this book and discover a new, healthier version of yourself. You will be introduced to an amazing world of natural therapies that will guide you towards your ultimate wellness. Additionally, this book can help you to lose weight, burn fat and gain vitality.

As for our enemy that we are planning to kill, *Señor* Cellulite, or *Señorita* Cellulite, depending on how big and strong it is, I can imagine what you're thinking now. Let me guess:

1. *Does it really work?*
2. *Oh no! This is another feel-good herbal book!*
3. *Yeah, right! I have tried everything and nothing has worked. Cellulite can't be cured! You have it, or you don't.*

I totally know how you feel. I felt really frustrated after spending a fortune on all of those expensive creams, lotions, peelings and other super *hyped* treatments that promised me they would cure cellulite in *x* days, weeks or months! Nothing seemed to work. I actually felt worse because not only did I end up as cellulite's victim but I also fell for all of those sales pitches promising miracles in dozens of bottles and substances filled with chemicals.

Luckily, my research coincided with my discovery of natural therapies, my personal and professional development and other big changes in my life. I began to study the holistic world, first as a hobby and then I decided to turn my passion into work. All of the therapies I studied and investigated, ranging from massage and oriental therapies to phytotherapy , homeopathy and even aromatherapy indicated the same statement: whatever sickness that is in your body is simply a sign of some other major imbalance that should be corrected.

The same applies to cellulite, as you will find out from this book. In fact, cellulite is just the tip of the iceberg. "Señor" Cellulite (or "Señorita" Cellulite) works for big mafias *like Low Energy Levels* and *Poor Circulation.* They mostly get paid by another corrupted mafia called: *Unhealthy Lifestyle.* We will analyze it all and try to get to the root of this unhealthy " corruption".

This book is a practical guide full of natural recipes that can help you fight off cellulite and keep it off forever if you stick to them. It's more about changing your lifestyle and maintaining the healthy way. It is not one of those x steps solutions that people normally get obsessed with before leaving on a vacation I am not judging, I have been there as well). The healthy and balanced lifestyle is more about a long-term commitment, not a one night stand if you get the comparison.

Throughout the book, I will provide you with certain specific recipes for phytotherapy, aromatherapy, natural food supplements etc. Those therapies are even faster and more efficient if you stick to the exact recipe that consists of different blends and precise measurements. Very often, people try to conduct certain treatments on their own, but without knowing which ingredients should be used together to create perfect synergy, it's possible to end up slowing down the whole process of cellulite reduction.

I will also explain some of the natural supplements that can be added to your diet, making you feel so much better, preventing food cravings, or choosing unhealthy foods. You will simply become more aware of your body - and what you feed it. It won't be a painful process, as we will first focus on what can be added to your daily routine, creating new healthy habits that I'm sure you will find enjoyable.

I will point to certain super foods that will keep your body well-nourished, and ensure that you thoroughly understand how important it is to eat healthily - and that doesn't have to be viewed as a sacrifice. You will definitely find this guide a bit different, as it tries to get to the root of the problem in a fully holistic way but it's written in a simple, conversational style.

You will learn which blends of herbs or essential oils to use and how to make them easy to apply. I will also mention other conditions that you can treat with the same natural ingredients. You will discover that you can take care of your body and mind at the same time and that you can get rid of cellulite very inexpensively. If you are concerned about animal testing then this is the book for you. My intention as a therapist is to promote aromatherapy and natural beauty products and I am strongly opposed to animal testing.

You will be surprised to see that my tips will also improve your general wellbeing, not only physically but also emotionally. The first results will be fast and the whole process can be a really pleasant ritual. It has worked for many of my clients, readers, friends and myself, and it will work for you as well. What makes this book a little bit different is that I provide you with different methods. The more you do the better but <u>you also have the flexibility</u> to choose whatever method suits you best. I tried to do my best not to preach to you and just tell you what to do. I prefer to provide you with certain tools that you can adapt and mould according to your lifestyle. Everyone is different; this is why I am not a big fan of so called health programs indicating the same thing for everyone. Of course I believe in those programs if they were designed in a tailored way for a person. I also think that this book will inspire you towards a really healthy lifestyle. This goal is always one of my main motivating forces to get me to writing.

Thanks again for purchasing my book, I hope you enjoy it! Don't forget to download the free, complimentary eBook: "Revolutionize Your Life with Alkaline Foods" as eating more alkaline (even if you don't follow a super strict alkaline diet) will surely help you on your holistic health and beauty journey. Download link: www.bitly.com/AlkalineMarta

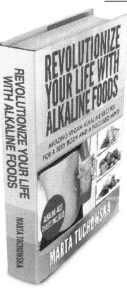

Disclaimer:
A physician has not written the information in this book. Although natural therapies are safe to use, if you suffer from any serious medical condition, are pregnant, or on medication you should **consult your physician first** to see if you can apply the natural therapies described in this book. It is also advisable that you visit a holistic health practitioner so that you can obtain a highly personalized treatment for your case. Most of natural therapies can be safely employed at the same time but it is still always recommended to consult your physician first.

All information in this book has been carefully researched and checked for factual accuracy. However, the author and publishers make no warranty, expressed or implied, that the information contained herein is appropriate for every individual, situation or purpose, and assume no responsibility for errors or omission. The reader assumes the risk and full responsibility for all actions, and the author will not be held liable for any loss or damage, whether consequential, incidental, and special or otherwise that may result from the information presented in this publication.

As for phytotherapy treatments, if you decide to try them please consult with your physician first as some of the herbal treatment may interfere with standard medications. It is also advisable to visit a specialized holistic health practitioner, phytotherapist, or an herbalist, that can design a treatment especially for you. The same applies to a diet and other natural therapies. The philosophy behind the holistic world is that everyone is different. As they say: *Different strokes, different folks.* In order for any natural treatment to be effective as well as 100% safe, one should seek a **professional advice with a qualified specialist**. Such advice can only be given after a detailed consultation with a holistic health practitioner of any of the therapies mentioned in this book or a naturopathic doctor. This book is for **educational and informative purposes** only.

Chapter 1

Holistic Therapies and Cellulite

Cellulite is basically subcutaneous fat that has been pushed into your dermis or the layer of skin beneath your epidermis, which is the outer layer. Your dermis contains your sweat glands, hair follicles, nerve receptors, and blood vessels. Underneath your dermis, there can be found two layers of subcutaneous fat which tends to protrude up into your dermis and create an orange-peel texture that is cellulite.

The fat seems bumpy because it pushes against your connective tissue, thus causing your skin to pucker. Cellulite commonly appears on the buttocks, back of the thighs, and hips. It also tends to get worse with age.

Causes of Cellulite

Cellulite can affect anyone, regardless of race, age, physique, and gender. However, it is more common in women than men. It does not only appear on people who are overweight. In fact, even thin people can have it.

Different factors can affect the production of cellulite, such as poor diet, slow metabolism, hormone changes, lack of physical activity, total body fat, dehydration, color and thickness of the skin, and even fad dieting (I prefer the word "lifestyle" as "diet" can be too stressful).

Genetics can also play a huge role in the formation of cellulite. If you come from a family with a history of cellulite, there is a high chance that you will have it too. Also, you should take note that the connective skin tissues of men and women have different structures. This is why women are more likely to develop cellulite than men.

12

The connective tissues are in the dermis and they are generally composed of water, elastic tissue, and collagen. It provides your dermis with a structure to help stabilize it. The connective tissue of women has a structure that is similar to a box and is separated by collagen columns.

Such arrangement lets fat push outwards towards the surface of the skin. This makes it seem like dimples. As for men, their connective tissue has more cross connections that tend to store the fat beneath the skin and allow it to expand inwards. Also, men have thicker epidermis, which is why their cellulite does not become easily noticeable.

OK, enough of boring theory. Now, let's dive into effective solutions...

Most cellulite books, or anti-cellulite books as we should call them, go into detail what cellulite is. However, I assume that if you are reading this book you already know all too well what it is and even where it can be found! Moreover, you are looking for solutions. In case you are reading this book out of curiosity because you became fascinated by the world of natural therapies (like I did a few years ago!), I assume you also want to take some action and read about natural therapies rather than twenty different definitions of cellulite.

Here comes my approach and simple anti-cellulite answers...

Think about a healthy body. There is balance, which means there is neither deficit nor overdose.

We should be happy and grateful that our bodies speak to us, as they always let us know when something is wrong. Don't simply look at cellulite as a beauty defect that must be eliminated. If you don't look at the actual causes and if you don't change certain habits, it will keep coming back. There is no quick fix, it is a process, but with the methods that I present to you, it will be very enjoyable, as you will discover many ways to take better care of your body. Wellness is a lifetime study and something that real wellness professionals never quit. You can never be healthy enough...

What will happen if you simply decide to focus on an effect? Well...

You will be spending a fortune on expensive beauty treatments and all o f those companies will be making money. Many of the chemical beauty products were tested on animals. If you like animals this is something you should keep in mind.

In all oriental medicine certain alarms that a body can give, are received as a blessing. It may sound a bit weird to Westerners as we hardly ever try to track the problem and get to the root of an illness or any imbalances that are present.

It is not a secret that people suffering from cellulite very often suffer from water retention, edema and irregular bowel movement. Cellulite marks might also appear from to hormonal changes or pregnancy.

Even slim people can suffer from cellulite. Cellulite and stretch marks can also appear after quick and intense weight-loss regimes (this was my story actually). Stress and lack of sleep very often lead to irregular eating patterns and unhealthier indulging that can later take their toll and appear as unwanted cellulite (again my story).

I have never been severely overweight (I had a few more kilos as a teen and in my early twenties and my weight would fluctuate from time to time,) and I thought that I was taking good care of myself. This is why I was surprised when I saw cellulite attacking my thighs. I thought that I was all ready for the summer and for the beach but it got me unexpectedly.

My first reaction was to go to my favorite beauty store and purchase a good amount of anti-cellulite creams and lotions. I also tried some pseudo-herbal diet supplements that only disagreed with my stomach and didn't really help me. Well, they did help people who sold them to make tons of money, but that's somewhat off topic. Perhaps you have realized that there is lots of money to be made in this so called beauty sector. Also, when it comes to purchasing supplements, I learned that it is really important to investigate the brand (the safest way is to purchase herbs and make your own blends, more on that later).

I was surprised I had cellulite because my mom never had it. It wasn't anything genetic in my case. But then I started to analyze my situation and came to a few conclusions:

1. Eating habits: yes, I thought I was eating healthily. I was convinced that after moving to Spain, I was sticking to a super healthy Mediterranean diet however; I did make a few mistakes. The Mediterranean diet is great if you also practice its relaxed philosophy and if you eat good quality, natural, nutritious meals prepared with love (sounds a bit new age I know!).

   I noticed that lack of time was the main culprit. Very often I would just have some super fried fast food ("tapas") and would still tell myself that I was eating a healthy, Southern-European diet. I didn't really have time to prepare my own meals (I was working and studying at the same time) and would eat out too often. There are not too many healthy restaurants or bars in Spain. I mean, the food is nice but not always healthy. It can be too fried and is not always natural. White bread is always used to make *bocatas* (sandwiches) and if you top this white bread with *tortilla de patatas* (potato complete- fried again) it is not the healthiest combination. Just my little remark on how the Mediterranean diet can mislead you sometimes if it is not done correctly. At the end of the day, I hardly ever had greens, salads or vegetable juices (BTW. these are great for weight loss and fat burn).

2. Stress Factor: at that time I had a really big goal: to quit my miserable 9-5 job in multilingual customer service and to become a massage therapist and wellness coach. This is why I was juggling my job, my studies, and my mini massage consultation to get my first clients and I just couldn't focus on the most important thing in this process: taking care of myself. Well, I did learn my lesson; I learned that health can never be the price for success and that if I want to be a wellness professional I first need to set an example for others. Imagine that you are a hairdresser or a stylist and your hair is horrible.

   Would you be likely to get any long-term clients or any clients at all?

   Imagine that you work in finances, let's say you are a financial consultant or a coach and you are broke. Would clients come to you? Or you are a dietician and you are overweight. A personal trainer that is in less shape than their clients. So yes, when it comes to the wellness sector, you must represent balance. Clients come to you as they seek balance. You must help them end the pain and help them to find balance. I knew I was getting out of balance. Cellulite was obviously one of the signs of it.

3. No exercise: before I got started on this wellness mission so as to change my job, I would go to the gym almost every day and take long trips in the mountains on the weekends. I had a regular workout routine. However, if you work and study, you will have very little time left. Add to it: getting started with a part-time business. As for weekends, I had to study. Moreover, I had to study anatomy and physiology in Spanish (I am not Spanish and it was a bit of a challenge). At the weekend I would also catch up with some workshops as well as some internet courses that I was doing. Again- even more

sedentary lifestyle all of a sudden. My body must have been freaking out.

OVERALL CONCLUSION: I was working myself out of balance. Even though I was happy and excited to pursue my wellness career, those couple of years of working and studying at the same time, were pretty hard. I was a workaholic.

-This is how Señor Cellulite knocked at my door. *Hey Marta, Can I please stay around?*

-I answered: *No, you can't stay here!*

At that time I was doing training in a really interesting form of a massage therapy, called lymphatic drainage (it is mentioned in the final chapters of this book). We were studying common conditions like slow circulation, edema and cellulite and learning how to alleviate them with manual therapy and naturopathy. As I mentioned before, my mother never had cellulite, but she has terrible varicose veins problems which I have inherited.

During this training I learned that common complaints like varicose veins, slow circulation, cellulite, edema and strae are very often interconnected. My teacher also knew a lot about naturopathy and I still admire her for everything she had taught me. She trained all over the globe so I was really lucky to be her student. She encouraged me to investigate phytotherapy. And so I went to check out my local herbalists' shop. I love all organic stores and herbal shops. I always have. Especially those little, cozy ones filled with natural fragrances that are very pleasant and healing. You become relaxed straight away. When I was a little girl I always thought it would be really 'cool' to work in one of those stores, hah! I still do.

My local herbalist was a really nice lady with amazingly strong curly hair, beautiful skin, and an impeccable, slim figure. I bet she was doing the real Mediterranean diet (I thought: wow it must be this herbal treatment thing, her appearance is the best business card for what she does!) I asked her if she had any phytotherapy treatments for cellulite. She looked at me not hiding her surprise and amazement and she asked me:

- *But...it's not for you, is it?*

I am quite tiny and slim I'm 5'5 and weigh 110 lbs) and I guess she thought that slim people don't need to worry about cellulite. Anyway, I'm not too sure what she thought, but she would look me up and down as if she was trying to measure my cellulite by scanning through my clothes! ☺

I said it was for me, and she was surprised. Still, she told me she had cellulite after losing massive weight and that phytotherapy helped her. She recommended a jar of already prepared mixed herbs. I grabbed them for only 5 euros (about 7 dollars, or 3 GBP). You must agree with that it was super cheap especially when compared to hundreds of (please fill with your local currency) spent on all those beauty products.

My friend, also called Marta, had spent even more money on all those magic cellulite treatments. After having her first baby she struggled both with weight gain and cellulite so she decided to join me. I was my very own guinea pig and at the same time I was her "coach".

Of course, it's not enough to drink herbal infusions, but the recipe that I share in phytotherapy chapter is very effective. It wasn't created by me or an herbalist who introduced it to me. It was actually invented by a medical doctor.

I changed my nutrition also. Well, I didn't actually change it but made it slightly healthier by doing an "anti-tapas detox". At that time I was also studying macrobiotic nutrition and discovered many foods that were new to me, like algae (Kombu, Wakame, Zori) and some superfoods like quinoa. I mainly focused on adding more nutrients to my diet so as to give my body some more well-deserved energy in a natural way.

As for Lymphatic Drainage, I had it done at least once a week. In a massage school, we would mostly practice on ourselves before getting the real patients, and in my free time I would swap my services with some of the girls (at least most of them were girls. If you are a guy and are looking for female company you should consider training in massage!) I met during the training. I was lucky to get treated to the lymphatic drainage therapy like twice a week.

I was also studying aromatherapy oils and natural spa treatments, something that I was testing on myself all the time. I learned that aromatherapy is much more therapeutic than we think and that it really is a holistic therapy.
I would massage the cellulite-affected areas with aromatherapy blends once or even twice a day. Even though, in my opinion, treating cellulite from the inside is the most important thing, aromatherapy can't be overlooked. It is a real pleasure for the senses and a really great holistic experience. Besides, who doesn't love spa treatments which, like many aromatherapy oils are soothing for the senses? Let's go for it! Relieving stress is definitely a good move if you want to kill cellulite. If your body is under too much stress, we can fall victims of emotional eating. By saying emotional eating, I mean indulging in certain foods that we all know are unhealthy but give us false enjoyment of temporary relief and feeds cellulite long-term (not judging, I have been there myself).

As I explained before, during that hectic era of pursuing my goals and ambitions (yes, I am a very ambitious person, sometimes maybe too much, but that's an area in which I am working to find balance) I didn't have time to hit the gym. By the time that I would finish school around eight or nine in the evening, get on the metro to catch the train back home, the gym would be already closed. Sometimes I would be lucky to get at least 15 minutes of swimming to refresh my mind (more than my body actually) but normally the pool was already closed when I was getting back home.

So I came up with a very simple solution for how to get my legs moving. First of all the most hated kind of work I have ever done is office work. I vow that I will never, ever do it again. But at that time it paid my rent and for my school. It was a blessing in disguise and a great way of achieving my long-term goals. Anyway, my legs and my whole body hate sitting which is exactly what you do when you work in an office. If you are Marta Tuchowska working in an office, then you take breaks constantly just to have some water or tea. Ask some of my ex-colleagues, they will tell you!

Even if you do take breaks, and even if you work part-time, if you are Marta Tuchowska, your legs won't feel great after an office work shift. It was too many hours in a sedentary position. Then you turn into a student and you attend your classes. Most of the people at the massage school that I was attending, were adults, from 25 to 50 years ole. Most of them were working in the mornings and attending classes in the afternoons or evenings (By the way, as you can see, it's never too late to pursue your dreams and change your career!).

And so during that period, Marta Tuchowska's legs had some really bad times. Sitting in a job, sitting in an anatomy class and then finally doing some massage (at least I could get some physical work there!) over the practical classes. Still in the end, I felt like the bad circulation would take its toll. If you have cellulite, you must have experienced this problem also; your legs are heavy and swollen and it feels like you can't move! Trust me, when you (and your legs) feel like that the least thing you want to do is to walk. Normally, you would feel like sitting. I had an excuse: the gym was closed- no 24-hour gyms. Still, I decided to take action and simply tried to skip a few metro stops and walk as much as possible.

When taking a 15 minutes break at work, or school, I would go and walk while drinking plenty of water. I then felt much more energized and therefore more motivated to continue my cellulite battle. Both I and my legs felt better. I knew that at least I was doing something. Instead of indulging in excuses, I found a solution. I know that it wasn't anything revolutionary but...do you know the feeling of when you take the stairs instead of taking the elevator? It takes some determination.

To round up my story, (sorry if it was too boring) I can tell you that I got rid of cellulite after three months. Very often I am asked how long it takes to get rid of cellulite using the methods I describe in this book. The answer will always be a bit inaccurate as it all depends on you really, but I guess that even if you have Señor Cellulite (yes, a big one), aiming for a few months to get rid of it can be a realistic goal. It's very hard for me to give you a definite answer in my book. Please contact me directly if it's something that is really on your mind (I am not offering any services here, just some free advice and inspiration). I would encourage you to focus on the process more than on the end result. In my efforts, I didn't know how much time it would take me to kill cellulite. Even though I managed to keep it off for a couple of years, I still maintain my anti-cellulite lifestyle. I know that I have this tendency as I am 32 years old now; my body is different than when I was 20(ah good times, but I like it now as well!). Anyway I am planning on looking good and healthy when I become 40, 50, and even 90 (that is, if I ever live as long as my grandpa who enjoyed 91 long years of life).

The reason I told you my boring story is to try to outline the mentality that you should have when trying to get rid of cellulite. If you still feel a bit confused please read on and ask yourself a few questions to see where you got the strategy wrong in the past.

Back to the American 24/7 gym I am sure I will check them out at some point.

Plus I would like to make a bold statement that one can always squeeze in a bit of exercise even in the busiest agendas. Everyone can take out 15 minutes a day, so instead of coming up with excuses, come up with solutions.

Let's focus on achieving our perfect body. Imagine you can wear anything you want. You look healthy. You feel light, you feel good and full of energy:

Are you ready to get started?

Your goal is to be healthy, feel healthy and look healthy. Therefore there is no way cellulite can stay where it is. You can get to the root of the problem, eliminate the causes of cellulite and say hello to your new, healthy and sexy body.

How you feel about your body attracts certain foods. Sounds weird? Then why do so many people always give up their diets and return to their unhealthy foods in exaggerated amounts that only make them feel awful about themselves and vicious circle goes on and on?

Whereas people who are already fit and healthy and full of energy, stick to their healthy foods and they can't imagine eating anything else... Avoiding fast food or junk food or processed food is not a sacrifice for them. The question is though - how to make this transition smooth, and easy?

Think healthy:

You only attract health and foods that fuel your body and mind. Anything else leads you far away from your goals.

As long as your body is in perfect balance there won't be anything like cellulite.

This means that your true objective should be:

22

I take care of my health truly and holistically!

Instead of just thinking: *No more cellulite, that's it but I am not going any deeper into what I should do to take care of my body!*

Think about cellulite as **an alarm** that is sounding because something is going wrong internally and creating these visible signs from the outside. As long as you understand that you will save time, money and energy, and you will get rid of your cellulite efficiently. It all starts on a cellular level.

The natural treatments that I explain in this book, will improve your body condition from the inside so you will have a perfect skin and a cellulite-free body. We will also focus on natural aromatherapy treatments to prepare, mixtures of oils to be applied to your skin. If you are new to aromatherapy it will be a great introduction for you and you will get addicted to it for sure.

If you already know a bit about aromatherapy it will take your experience to a more holistic and advanced level.

As for Señor cellulite, the lesson to be learned in this chapter is to put health before the cellulite problem. The same when it comes to weight loss. In one of my other books about motivation I say how important it is to put wellness before weight loss.

Having said that we can get to the root of the problem!

Adios cellulite!

Chapter 2

Your Friends and Your Enemies

You probably already know what to avoid, but you might be having difficulty finding out exactly how to do it. How do I overcome these food cravings?
You need to find your weak points: is it chocolate, sweets, sugar? Is it bread, alcohol, croissants, ice- cream, fast-food or kebabs?

It might seem like a sacrifice at first, but after a while it will become a shadow from the past. A healthy body that doesn't lack any nutrients and that is well maintained by healthy nutrition does not seek these foods. If you have those constant cravings for unhealthy foods, this constant desire to eat, then try to see it as an internal body alarm.

Your body tries to tell you something: *Feed me with good food! I lack nutrients*!

This is where most diets go wrong. They first tell you what to avoid and they try to make it quick. You manage to eliminate wrong foods from your diet however you don't add anything new that can actually make permanent changes.

My point is: By adding some foods into your diet to begin with, even though they may seem a little weird to you at first (i.e. herbs and other natural supplements), you will find it easier to avoid the bad foods. It's as easy as that.

For example, I do have chocolate or ice-cream once in a while, the same with *an* occasional pizza or eating out, but only when I choose the moment to have them, usually as a special treat. They don't choose me as a victim, I choose them. But it is no longer a craving and it is always controllable. Body and mind form an inseparable part.

For now though, I only want you to find the main culprits in your diet. Be honest with yourself, but don't get too obsessed. No guilt-trips.

List all the foods that you know you should avoid: Too much caffeine, soft drinks, alcohol, chocolate, supermarket meat, fast food, sweets, etc. In fact all foods that are readymade, packaged and not fresh are not helping either.

Keep the list whilst you're reading this book and try to switch to healthy alternatives.

You might also like to create a vision board. Put up a picture of the ideal body that you want to have and beside it list your top 10 food enemies. Whenever you get lazy or get some 'enemy' foods craving, just ask yourself:

Is it worth it? How much time and money have I already invested in reading, researching and actually trying to change something about my body?

Now it's time to change it once and for all.

It is all part of a process that you are now undertaking. So don't give up! Slight changes may be needed, but done persistently; every day will bring more benefits in the long run. Jumping from one method to another or giving up after a week or so can only lead you back to where you were before.

Be patient and persistent and stick to the natural way. It will surely become your lifestyle. Let's do it step-by-step.

Chapter 3

Caffeine and Cellulite

It might seem like a huge sacrifice for you at first but abusing coffee won't help to get rid of cellulite. Caffeine will further retain water and some toxins will not be flushed out properly. You have probably tried different anti-cellulite creams with caffeine – caffeine used as an ingredient to be applied externally can be very effective. However, it won't help when you drink too much of it. Not to mention other imbalances in your body that it can cause.

If you know you abuse caffeine (coffee, black tea, or other caffeinated drinks, for example some energy drinks), you should start planning to quit, not only because you don't want to have any more cellulite signs but also because you want to gain higher energy levels and more awareness of how to take care of your body. You don't have to be radical; you can have coffee occasionally, but don't abuse it. To cut a long story short: coffee for cellulite? Yes, but on your body— not in your mouth.

This is how you can use coffee on your body:

As a shower scrub

Place the granules in a bowl and add little bit of vegetable oil (the oil must be cold-pressed), e.g. sweet almond oil, rapeseed oil, avocado oil. Stir the mixture for a few minutes and scrub cellulite-affected areas. The aroma of coffee is also very awakening for your senses, sometimes our body doesn't really want an intake of coffee it's just the aroma that our mind wants so desperately. Apply the scrub on the cellulite affected areas.

As Body Lotion

You can grind some dry coffee granules and add this powder to your body lotion (the more natural your lotion is - the better). The only drawback is that it may stain your clothes, so make sure that if you use it at night time you wear an old night-dress.

How coffee or black teas in exaggeration worsen the cellulite problem?

Excessive caffeine consumption will make your body de-hydrated.The most effective way of treating cellulite and successfully removing it, is to make use of the body's natural ability to flush out toxins. When the body holds water there is no way in the world that it will be able to do this. Your body will try to prevent your system from becoming totally de-hydrated by holding the water internally when the water you put inside your body is insufficient. Then, not only can the cellulite get worse, but you will feel really tired and not at all inspired to make any positive changes like implementing a healthy diet or workout regime. Again, it is not solely caffeine that provokes cellulite, it doesn't really cause it, but its consumption will aggravate the problem.

After reading this and gaining more awareness I suggest you grab a glass of fresh water and add some freshly squeezed organic lemon juice. Smell its fresh scent and think about all the cells in your body that are being hydrated and how your system is slowly getting rid of toxins. Breathing in and out in a conscious manner will also give you more energy and speed up the process of detoxification. Make sure that your body is always well-hydrated the way it needs it. These methods may seem to be very obvious but it's surprising how many times we forget to apply them.

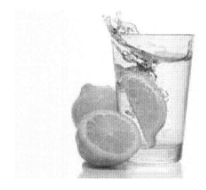

I am not trying to tell you to stop drinking coffee at all, unless you really want to try it. Personally, I treat myself to a cup of coffee every now and then, but I don't rely on it for energy. I also make sure that the coffee that I drink is organic. The cheap, industrial coffee is full of chemicals and toxins that can be very detrimental to your health. And yes, if you are suffering from cellulite, it can aggravate the problem.

More about caffeine:

Caffeine increases the heart rate, elevates blood pressure and provokes anxiety, muscular tension, irritability, indigestion, insomnia, decreased immunity, lack of energy, emotional imbalances, gastrointestinal problems, sugar swings, nutritional deficiencies, (females are especially affected), osteoporosis, menopausal problems, adrenal exhaustion, chronic and fatigue. It can even contribute to premenstrual syndrome and make it more painful and annoying! Do you really want to deprive your body of even more iron even?

There are many coffee substitutes that can help you reduce cellulite and gain more energy levels and health in the long run. There are so many of them you can actually pick and choose the one that suits you best.

I suggest you try some coffee substitutes instead. You can also try black tea, but remember that it also contains high levels of caffeine and so when abused, it can react quite similarly as coffee. However if not too strong, and with a slice of lemon and ginger in it, it's a great detoxifying drink

Green Tea

It has much less caffeine than black tea or coffee and it is a very powerful antioxidant. You need antioxidants in your diet, both if your goal is cellulite reduction as well as if you wish to improve your energy levels. It is also very efficient for weight-loss treatments.

Red Tea

Its properties are very similar to those of green tea, but it can also contribute further to the burning of fat. Another Red Tea health benefit is the ability to lower cholesterol levels. Drinking two cups of Red Tea every day for three weeks opens capillaries and helps maintain normal blood pressure. It is also great for the digestion.

Rooibois
It is a great option if you can't stand the taste of green or red tea! Personally, I love green tea but some people don't like the bitter taste of it. Rooibois tastes very nice, a little bit sweet, it is actually caffeine-free and helps stimulate venous circulation and therefore toxin elimination. This is why it results in a great remedy for cellulite.

Furthermore, it contains several minerals that are vital to maintaining perfect health. These include:

-Magnesium: essential for the nervous system
-Calcium: essential for strong teeth and bones
-Zinc: important for metabolism
-Iron: important for helping blood & muscles distribute oxygen

Drinking two cups of Rooibois every day will make you feel nicely energized and more alert. You will start noticing these changes after only a few days.

Kukicha: The tea of three years
A lovely tea with almost no theine; it can even be given to children for breakfast. It provides us with a great quantity of natural calcium, which is absorbed by our body and fixed to our bones. It has re-mineralizing and alkalizing effects and detoxifies the body, which is very important when it comes to cellulite reduction.

The main beneficial effect of Kukicha tea comes from its strong alkalizing power. This drink helps to alkalize body tissues and fluids, balancing their acid levels and preventing multiple diseases.

Include Kukicha tea with your breakfast or mid-afternoon snack, and you will obtain a natural energy drink.

White Tea

Contains virtually no theine and has strong antioxidant effects that will speed up your metabolism. White tea has many other benefits to offer: it reduces blood sugar and helps prevent and alleviate the symptoms of diabetes. It reduces stress and increases energy.

Start now by choosing your favorite substitutes and you will be able to create effective cellulite treatments from within. If you are planning on doing a coffee detox, you should be able to regain your natural energy within a week or two. Just by quitting coffee or at least reducing it, you will notice a positive effect and the cellulite marks will diminish a bit. You will also improve your circulation naturally and prepare your body to fight cellulite effectively.

Chapter 4

Phytotherapy and Herbs

This chapter is very easy to understand and to apply as it contains some effective herbal recipes. You can either ask your local herbalist to prepare the blends for you (it is important to stick to the proportions outlined) or try to choose at least 3 of the herbs mentioned in this chapter and experiment in preparing various infusions depending on your taste preferences. It doesn't have to be painful and you shouldn't force yourself into drinking something that you can't stand.

The option I recommend though is it to stick to the exact recipe as it will be much more effective. It is something that you can get started on immediately and then you can focus on other strategies like what to avoid in your diet and what to add. This is what I did-I used the phytotherapy recipe in the blend that I explain in this chapter. Very often, the herbs are more effective when working together, with other herbs. The art and science of phytotherapy comes down to knowing how to mix them to make the treatments more effective.

Now, I am not a certified phytotherapist, I am just really interested in herbs and I keep investigating and always involve myself in workshops and do lots of research. Whenever seeking a specific treatment, I consult with a qualified phytotherapist. I don't know if you realize, but it's a life-long study. Real phytotherapists study for years just to get started. And they never actually stop studying.

As I said before, it is normally easier to start with adding some new foods, supplements or herbs and then focus on eliminating the enemies. This is how you can fight the unhealthy foods cravings: first add some new and healthy stimulus to your body and then you will find it much easier to eliminate your enemies. Your body will feel stronger and much more balanced.

When I first started using herbs to eliminate cellulite I began noticing some really positive changes in my body and also in my mind. I would wake up with more energy and the water retention was gone. My mind felt much more focused and I just found it a lot of easier to carry on with my healthy lifestyle and simply getting back on track.

If you have any friends or family suffering from cellulite, water retention, low energy levels, or even slow bowel movements, you can recommend this wonderful herbal recipe to them. It's also great for general body & mind detox and is a wonderful, non-caffeine infusion. If you can't stand its bitter taste you can sweeten it with stevia.

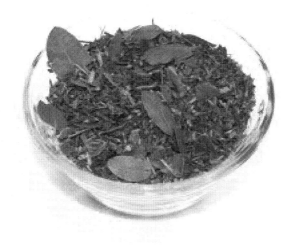

The herbal treatment should be followed for at least a month. Drink 1- 2 cups of a prepared herbal infusion a day. Use 1- 2 tablespoons of the mixture. Ask your herbalist to prepare the following herbs for you and mix them in a jar. They will be ready for you to be turned into delicious infusions. All herbs listed below should be mixed in proportions as specified.

For one jar:

Fucus Vesiculosus: 20 gr
Oxiacanta Crataegus: 10 gr
Flipendula ulmaria: 15 gr
Butula Alba: 15 gr
Fraxinus Excelsior: 10 gr
Verbena Offic: 10 gr
Equisetum: 10 gr

Of course you or your herbalist can figure out the ratio of ingredients and adjust the quantity. Show them this recipe, I am sure they will like it.
The total of 90gr yield of this blend will be enough for the one month treatment.
If you are undergoing any other treatments (even if they are natural), please consult your doctor or a qualified herbalist first. <u>Abstain from using these herbs if you are pregnant or lactating.</u>

Let's have a look at each herb separately, you might also be interested in creating your own blend, depending which herbs you prefer. It's up to you if you want to modify the recipe slightly and make it more personalized.

The reason why so many people either get put off or attracted to certain herbal treatments is because of their taste. It will be easier for you to follow a natural treatment that is also enjoyable for you. Try some of the herbs and decide for yourself:

Fucus vesiculosus

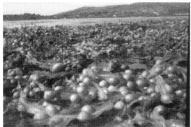 **Fucus is my favorite of the whole mix!**

This is a type of seaweed (North and Baltic Seas as well as Atlantic and Pacific Oceans) with the common name is *bladder wrack*, also known as *black tang, rockweed, bladder fucus, sea oak, black tany, cut weed* and *rock wrack*.

It is used for the whole range of medical conditions, like iodine deficiencies and others related to thyroid disorders like underactive thyroid and goiter.
It is also used in treating obesity and hardened arteries, balancing cholesterol and glucose levels.

Famous for its anti-inflammatory properties, fucus vesiculosus is given to people with arthritis, rheumatism, and joint pain. As a topical treatment this herb has been used to alleviate painful skin diseases, burns, aging skin, and insect bites. Finally, fucus vesiculosus has also been tested as a treatment for pre-menopausal women and others with urinary tract infections.

Why is it effective in reducing cellulite? Numerous studies have shown that thanks to high contents of the phytochemical fucoidan can reduce fat and stimulate microcirculation. It also reduces excess fluids in body tissues.

It's taste is not something that most of the people would enjoy, which is why I always recommend mixing it with other herbs or taking it in the form of capsules; they contain the plant but in form of dry powder. Personally I think that nothing can beat a delicious herbal infusion (you know how I love the taste of herbs!) but I must recognize the fact that in this day and age, phytotherapy capsules are much more practical. I have used them also, but very often I would break the capsule and just try to get some powder as the capsule is definitely not natural. Also, if you want to use herbs in form of capsules, tablets and other supplements that are ready to take on the go, make sure that you research the brand. The market is full of falsely labeled 'natural' stuff and false claims. I'd rather not get into this, as my blood pressure is raising just at the thought of people selling seemingly natural things which can be even harmful.

Oxciacanta

This herb has many therapeutic indications, like hypertension, angina, and peripheral vascular disorders. What really should interest you is that oxciacanta is a powerful antioxidant and has some strong lipid regulating properties. All the herbs and foods that are rich in antioxidants are very useful in cellulite elimination.

Most people would consider its taste pleasant. Try it yourself to see whether you fit in that category.

You have probably realized by now, that all the plants have more than just one therapeutic property; it will work the same in aromatherapy as well as in homeopathy. However, remember that different doses are used for different problems. Normally when you acquire some therapeutic herbs, your herbalist will give you specific advice, or if you buy ready-made infusions, these packets will have recommended doses that you should always stick to. Too much of something, even if natural, can also do harm.

Let's have a look at the rest of anti- cellulite herbs.

Flipendula ulmaria

Its common name is Meadowsweet seeds and it is known for being analgesic, anti-inflammatory, antipyretic, diuretic and anti-cellulite. Interestingly enough, this herb has been used for natural pain treatment and to reduce fever. Small amounts of the meadowsweet root can be used to get rid of headaches; this is believed to be effective because of the aspirin-like components present in the herb. A tisane prepared from the meadowsweet flowers can render comfort to individuals affected by flu.

It is also called "sacred plant of the druids" because of its multiple healing properties; it formed part of many of their rituals.

For a person seeking a natural anti-cellulite herbal treatment, this plant can really work miracles as it is a powerful diuretic as well as depurative, anti-toxin and anti-cellulite. It has got a pleasant taste and flavor and so including it as a regular herbal drink can be a really nice and healthy ritual.

Betula Alba

Its common name is Birch bark tea. It helps clean and purify the skin and is also used for blood detoxification.

It is commonly used for hair loss treatments as it prevents hair loss and stimulates hair growth. This infusion can be applied as a hair tonic.
Thanks to its diuretic cleansing action, it eliminates toxins and is a must for anti-cellulite treatments. It is also very helpful in weight loss treatments. Its natural, herbal-sweet taste makes *betula alba* infusions a very nice experience.

37

Fraxinus Excelsior

It is also known as *ash*, this plant is perhaps a little bit less known, but should still be included in natural anti-cellulite treatments.
The leaves have diuretic, diaphoretic and purgative properties, and are famous for their medical properties. It is considered a great remedy for dropsy and obesity. The taste is bitter and it may take a while to get used to it.

Verbena Officinalis

Also called **Common Vervain** or **Common Verbena,** this herb strengthens the nervous system, de-stresses the body and mind and helps with digestion. It is rich in **flavanoids** which are really powerful antioxidants that help the body to get rid of toxins and contribute to cellulite reduction drastically.

They have also been used for nervous disorders and are still used by herbalists for soothing anxiety and stress and promoting relaxation and sleep. They have sedative and astringent properties.

Equisetum

More commonly referred to as horsetail, this infusion is a well-known, natural and easy to use herbal remedy with a really pleasant taste. It has amazingly strong properties to detoxify the body and the mind and to eliminate toxins. It prevents water retention and can even burn fat; this is why it is a common supplement in weight loss diets. What is also very interesting is that horsetail infusions promote healthy skin and hair; they reinforce microcirculation and are full of minerals. It can be very helpful if you want to have healthy and strong nails and get rid of acne or oily skin conditions.

If you suffer from stress, chronic migraines etc, include a horsetail infusion in your daily routine. Its high levels of potassium, magnesium, calcium, iron and zinc will help you fight stressful situations effectively. Equisetum infusion is another great coffee substitute. As I mentioned before, coffee only causes you to flush out all of these important minerals, while retaining the toxins in at the same time. Instead, we want to have it the other way round so we can be full of energy.

Enjoy your herbal treatments!

Chapter 5

Aromatherapy and Spa Treatments

I can guarantee that you will absolutely love this therapy. Since I discovered aromatherapy and began my training as an aromatherapist, I have given up all the chemical cosmetics and beauty products. I started using and preparing my own aromatherapy oil blends for beauty, health and wellness. At first I thought that it would be extremely time-consuming but actually, it isn't. Another benefit of using aromatherapy, whether for beauty, health, wellbeing or relaxation, is that you will save lots of space on your bathroom shelves. All the aromatherapy treatments are multifunctional and so it is a never-ending story.

In the previous chapter I mentioned different herbs and how rich they are in certain substances than can help you burn fat, fight headaches or eliminate cellulite.

Aromatherapy, just like phytotherapy, is also about herbs. The only difference is that aromatherapy treatments are normally applied topically, via massage. There are also exceptions to this rule (The French School of aromatherapy, called medical aromatherapy or *aromatology*, also advocates the oral use of the essential oils) but it won't be covered in this book as it is not normally used in the spa world nor for anti-cellulite treatments. I wanted to let you know that such an approach also exists and that it forms part of many naturopathic treatments.

So what are the basics of Aromatherapy?
As a massage therapist, very often I get asked about massage oils etc. I noticed that many people get confused when it comes to essential oils and vegetable oils. I have been there

myself; some time ago and it was also a mystery to me. Let me explain it to you:

Essential oils- those are extracted from different plants and can be diluted in cold-pressed vegetable oils and used in various health and beauty treatments depending on their properties. Aromatherapy oils are rich in various substances that can help you fight a whole range of conditions on a mental, emotional and physical level.

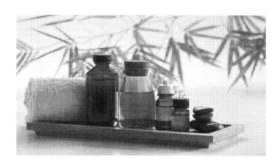

Some basics about aromatherapy essential oils
Essential oils shouldn't be applied in their pure form because they may cause an allergic reaction. This is why they must be previously diluted in good quality base oil.
Another thing is - contrary to their name - they are not oily at all. Although they are called essential oils, I would prefer to call them essences, since this term makes it easier to understand what aromatherapy is about.

It is very easy to prepare your own blends and it is not necessary to follow my recipes. You can just prepare your mix to fight cellulite, burn fat or stimulate circulation, store it in a dark, glass bottle and use it as a body lotion. All you need to do is to pick up a few essential oils from the list below, as well as one vegetable oil (also called carrier oil or base oil).

This will be your new aromatherapy ritual (which I hope you will enjoy!).

41

Certain aromatherapy oils have some really powerful anti-cellulite and fat-burn properties but they are also really multifunctional so you can use them in other treatments too. Creating your natural anti-cellulite oil blend is a fast, natural and cheap alternative for expensive creams and lotions. Moreover, you can use the same oils for other beauty treatments.

Juniper Essential Oil

Its smell is not the most appealing for some people. Others find it quite nice and others just bearable. That said, it is not only about the aromas, it's mostly about the properties that the oils have. Juniper oil can work miracles for water retention and cellulite. It has some really strong anti- oxidant properties as well. When you apply it on to your skin, it will be absorbed and will enter your system via the circulation.

It is recommended for people wanting to detox or people undergoing hangover symptoms (yes!). It reduces fat and cellulite in a really fast way and therefore I truly recommend that you add it to your mixture.
If you tend to suffer from bad circulation, edema, water retention, obesity, o r chronic fatigue etc. the juniper essential oil should be included in your aromatherapy blends.

Other properties: Add a few drops to your shampoo. This oil stimulates hair growth and if used on a regular basis, can improve your hair condition naturally.

Lemon, Grapefruit, Orange, Mandarin Essential Oils

These essential oils are relatively cheap and very easy to get hold of. The high content of vitamin C contributes to reducing cellulite and striae while also improving the skin tone.

Very important: Avoid using these oils before being exposed to the sun as they are **photo-toxic**.

Other properties: The fresh citric scent is recommended to combat headaches, stress and low energy levels, as well as mental exhaustion. Apply a few drops on your pillow or to your inner wrists. You can also dilute it in a vegetable oil and massage into your neck and temples.
Add a few drops of lemon essential oil to your shampoo or conditioner, for extra shine.

Geranium

This oil works well for water retention conditions, especially tired legs. It acts as natural lymphatic drainage by stimulating lymphatic and venous circulation and eliminating toxins, therefore reducing cellulite visibly. On a mental and emotional level, it helps to fight tension headaches and has energizing properties. I first tried this oil in massage school and it has become one of my favorites ever since. I use it on a regular basis. If your legs feel tired after a long day at work, a quick geranium oil massage is something that your legs will be truly grateful for. I also use geranium oil for my skin which tends to be oily sometimes.

Other properties: If you add one drop of geranium essential oil to your face cream, you will be able to regulate sebum secretion while hydrating your skin at the same time. Since geranium is one of the very few essential oils that has adapting properties, it can be also used if your skin is dry, and it will regulate the natural sebum to re-hydrate it. Before using this oil on your face (even if it's only one drop diluted in your facial cream) please test it on your wrists first. If your skin is really sensitive it might turn red and itchy.

Fennel

Fennel oil has a wonderful, spicy-herbal smell. It is famous for its diuretic effect, works as natural lymphatic drainage, helps to disperse cellulite and reduce fat. It will give you a feeling of light relief, as if your body weighs less!

Other properties: The fennel oil offers many benefits for the mind as well: it provides courage and strength in the face of adversity. It has a cleansing and toning effect on the skin, helping with bruises, overly oily skin and will help to fight wrinkles at the same time. Simply add a drop to your every day face cream or face tonic.

Additional info: fennel tea is amazing as well. Read this article on my blog to learn more: www.holisticwellnessproject.com/blog/health-wellness/health-benefits-of-fennel-tea/

Cypress

This essential oil has really fresh, forest-like aroma. Not only is it diuretic but also a vasoconstrictor, meaning that it alleviates varicose veins. It is a great remedy for water retention. On a mental level it is a great remedy for nervous or angry people as it has a highly-soothing effect. It also alleviates menopause problems.

Other properties: This oil is said to encourage creativity, perfect for writers and artists. On a physical level, it is a natural cold remedy. Simply massage your chest and neck with a bit of cypress oil (of course, never pure. Check the dilatations that follow) or use it for inhalations.

Cinnamon

Did you know that this oil is also widely employed as an aphrodisiac...?
It is known as a stimulant, both for the body and mind. Its main components will not be able to eliminate cellulite efficiently, but because it is great for sluggish circulation and lymphatic system dysfunctions, it should definitely be included in you aromatherapy blend to fight cellulite.

Other properties: Cinnamon can help you to overcome nervousness, exhaustion and it is also great oil for rheumatic pain relief. It is especially nice for the winter time as it also prevents colds and strengthens the immune system.

Ylang-ylang

Ylang-ylang is also an aphrodisiac. Its smell is strong and flowery, though some people might find it too heavy. It has a strong hydrating effect on the skin. Again, just like cinnamon oil, when used on its own, it won't work miracles on cellulite, but when mixed with other oils, will further increase hydration and reduce striae. It has great anti-frustration properties for the mind and emotions and increases motivation.

Other properties: it is a strong aphrodisiac (apparently more so for females than males), natural hair tonic (dilute in a vegetable oil and massage your scalp at least an hour before washing your hair), and it is great for treating acne and oily skin.

How to use essential oils:

We are going to follow the simple aromatherapy rules that are native to the British School of aromatherapy. While many other approaches exist and they are all correct, this one is great for beginners and it is normally used in spas.

You will need at least one of the vegetable based oils. Make sure they are natural and pure: sweet almond oil, hazelnut oil, olive oil, coconut, calendula, apricot, avocado, grape seed, or jojoba.

The cheapest option is sweet almond oil. Almond oil is actually my favorite massage oil. Quality at an affordable price is what everyone is looking for these days.

If you are looking for easily-absorbed oils you can go for apricot kernel oil; it is also recommended for facials due to its light consistency.

The base oil normally employed in anti-cellulite treatments is hazelnut oil, as it is famous for its penetrating and nourishing properties. This is how you can make sure that all the essential oils you put in a mixture will be absorbed quickly and efficiently.

Choose at least 4 essential oils with strong anti-cellulite and anti fluid-retention properties. You can also add some cinnamon or ylang-ylang oil to make it spicier.

These are the proportions to stick to, more or less:
-For 15 ml of the carrier oil, use about 6 or 7 drops of essential oil(s) (in total if you are adding more than one oil)
-2ml carrier oil use 1 drop of essential oil
-1 tablespoon is more or less 15 ml.

For example if you are using a 50 ml bottle filled with vegetable (base) oil, then around 25 drops of essential oil(s) should be added for the blend to be effective.

Apply the blend twice or 3 times a day on the affected areas, using energetic, friction-like movements and kneading the area.

A slight, pain-provoking aggression should be employed in the rubbing movements.

Commit to your aromatherapy home spa. You will be surprised at its multifunctional properties.

As for aromatherapy for cellulite as well as for massage treatments, they are all great and all natural additions that can stimulate the process of killing cellulite. However, as I already said and will repeat again: *it all starts on the cellular level.*

Remember that the real changes come from inside!

Aromatherapy oils for cellulite are also great, natural, moisturizing treatments. The biggest hurdle is to become committed to them on a regular basis. Here is what I do: once a week, I prepare a small bottle of my aromatherapy blend and I keep it in my gym bag. Since I exercise and then shower at the gym, this aromatherapy ritual now forms part of the whole process. It's all about creating simple systems to be nicely organized and incorporate aromatherapy into your life.

You can do the same at home- prepare your blend once a week (this is how you can save time and just make this whole process a bit more automatic) and use it as your holistic body lotion. You will also do a big favor to your pockets!

I also get asked about sponges and peelings. To be honest, I never actually committed to regular peelings myself. But if you can do it and massage cellulite areas with a special sponge and also do a good natural peeling (see the previous chapter about coffee) the only thing you have to lose is cellulite. It is a great, additional anti-cellulite treatment and it will also prepare your skin for oils.

Finally, another natural and really nice, additional treatment is hydro massage. Maybe you have a Jacuzzi at home (I don't), if not check out your local gym, or pool or even spa for hydro massage. Again, don't expect miracles with this one alone; it is a simple, <u>additional strategy</u> that requires no effort which is the reason why I included it.

Chapter 6

Foods that Eliminate Cellulite

We will now have a closer look at what should be included in your diet and what should be avoided. All these new, fresh foods and natural supplements will make the 'going healthy' transition smooth, easy and enjoyable.

Rome wasn't built in a day so try to take your time and have fun with the process of going healthier.

Cellulite is normally connected to different health conditions like venous insufficiency, varicose veins, phlebitis, ulcers, edema, water retention as well as premenstrual syndrome. If you want to get rid of cellulite and prevent the above-mentioned conditions, you need to understand that it all comes down to …taking proper care of **your veins and your circulation**. While following your new, healthy diet not only can you fight the cellulite, but also you invest in your health, meaning that you will lower the risks of suffering from any of the conditions I have just mentioned.

The venous system functions to direct the oxygen-poor blood and the toxins from the muscles and tissues towards the heart. Any dysfunctions that cause the metabolic system to slow down will make the bodily cells and tissues accumulate toxins.

The factors that further slow down your metabolism are:

1. Sedentary work/ lifestyle

2. Hot temperatures

3. Poor muscle tone

4. Abusing alcohol, caffeine, chocolate, spices

5. Too much time in the standing position (jobs like shop assistant, hairdresser, etc)

6. Too many fried foods

7. Heavily processed foods (or just 'processed foods')

Remember that all the circulatory problems, when neglected, can lead to serious problems, like e.g. phlebitis.

I have prepared a really general outline so that you can analyze your nutritional habits. I don't know where you are standing now, but from my own experience I know that there is always something that can be improved.

Foods and nutrients that you need:

Flavanoids

I have mentioned this term before. Flavanoids are cellulite's big enemy as they are rich in antioxidants (it is important to keep this in mind if you have a high-stress level lifestyle or if you want to detoxify). They also protect the venous structure and speed up toxin elimination and prevent excessive inflammation throughout your body. Sources of flavanoids include: apples, apricots, blueberries, pears, raspberries, strawberries, black beans, cabbage, onions, parsley and tomatoes.

Vitamin C and other antioxidants

Flavanoids work together with vitamin C, which has the same properties, its effect is both preventative and curative.

Many fresh fruits and vegetables contain relatively high amounts of vitamin C. Here are some of the top foods for getting this very important nutrient into your diet: papaya, strawberries, broccoli, brussels sprouts, oranges, lemons, tomatoes and peaches.

Make sure that the fruits and vegetables you eat are organic.

Silicon

Silicon is known to be needed for synthesis of elastin and collagen and can make the skin's surface perfect and smooth. It is found in many fibrous foods such as celery, peppers, carrots, potatoes, unrefined grains (for example quinoa, beets as well as in hemp leaves, nettles leaves and horsetail (tremendous source). Other herbal sources of silicon include alfalfa, chickweed, corn silk, dandelion, red raspberry, oat straw and stinging nettle. Don't forget that silicon is also found in shiny fruits and veggies such as red peppers, tomatoes and cucumbers. I recommend that you try some algae as well (e.g. spirulina or chlorella).

Omega 3

It acts in perfect synergy with other antioxidants, eliminating the risk of phlebitis and increasing overall energy levels and improving memory. It also lowers the amount of lipids (fats such as cholesterol and triglycerides) circulating in the bloodstream. Make sure that you eat foods like: sardines, salmon, flax seeds and walnuts to promote healthy cell membranes and reduce cellulite.

Vitamins B9, B12, B6 and Magnesium

The lack of those vitamins (as well as magnesium imbalances) can slow down the metabolism; this is why it is essential to make sure you incorporate foods rich in those vitamins and magnesium in your diet. Remember that abusing caffeine depletes your body of magnesium and inhibits iron absorption.

By increasing the intake of those vitamins, not only will you feel more energized and focused, but you will also be in much better mood; all you need if you're looking for a healthy and balanced lifestyle.

Go for foods like: almonds, bananas, sunflower seeds, dark leafy greens, fresh and dried fruits, organic eggs, chia seeds and quinoa.

Zinc and Vitamin A

Zinc and Vitamin A are necessary for wound healing and work great for striae reduction.
Try to include foods like: seafood, roasted pumpkin and squash seeds, nuts, carrots, and dark leafy greens.

Magnesium

If there is magnesium deficiency there is more sodium inside the cell and sodium tends to retain water, this is why magnesium is indispensible if you wish to fight cellulite, fluid retention and feel more energized. Magnesium rich foods include: bananas, avocados, dried fruits, fish, beans and lentils. You may also start adding alkaline salts to your water.

Check out my website: www.HolisticWellnessProject.com for some recommendations.

Potassium

Potassium lowers water retention and premenstrual tension. Reduces striae and cellulite marks and is necessary for optimal energy levels.

Go for foods like: apricots, white beans, spinach, salmon, bananas, sweet potatoes, and white mushrooms.

If you are not in habit of eating organic, healthy and nutritious foods, start planning your transition. It's not only about eliminating cellulite, it's about being healthy and energetic. As soon as you start eating what I call 'Real foods' you will be amazed at the results and your increased zest for life! I believe in nutritious eating and I reject all fad diets or any diets that out way too much strain on your mind and soul or even go as far as encouraging you to starve yourself. I always try to base my approach on balance and common-sense.

You can keep discovering and adding some new super foods regularly. Try to add something new to your diet every day or at least every week. Small changes will create big results.

Quinoa

This crop is native to the Andes. It can be great pasta replacement. Quinoa is a super grain (gluten-free) that will make your stomach feel full and prevent you from feeling food cravings. It offers the whole range of health benefits as it is packed with many vitamins and minerals including:

-Heart-healthy mono-unsaturated fat (oleic acid) and omega-3 fatty acid (a-linolenic acid)

-Antioxidant phytonutrients called flavonoids

-Essential minerals including manganese, magnesium, iron, phosphorus, potassium, calcium, zinc, copper and selenium

-Vitamins: B1, B2, B3, B6, B9, E,

- a great source of fiber

For example, if you have a craving for pasta with pesto (I love that dish, just like all the pastas and pizzas. I have lived in Italy and I've tried it all!), try to use quinoa instead of pasta, prepare a home-made pesto (so here we avoid preservatives) and if you want to go even further and make it more vegan, you can use almond powder instead of cheese.

Check out this article on my blog to learn more about quinoa (recipes included): www.holisticwellnessproject.com/blog/health-wellness/health-benefits-of-quinoa/

Amaranth

Amaranth is another super grain from South America. A source of all dietary protein and fat, anti-inflammatory properties, it is also called 'natural weight-loss food'. It is especially rich in iron and complex carbohydrates which make it a super food: healthier for you and great for any weight-loss diet as well.
I love to start my day with amaranth. A great breakfast idea: amaranth porridge! Use vegan milk (unless you really like cow's milk, some people do and it works fine for them but personally, I always use vegan milks: rice, soy, almond, oat milk just to name a few). Spice it up with some cinnamon and add some blueberries. You will keep your energy levels high and your body will be nicely nourished (not only fed).

Also, as I explained earlier, if you tend to suffer from cellulite, you need to take good care of your circulation.

Millet

It is very similar to couscous. It is one of the few grains that are alkalizing. It boosts metabolism and has a high antioxidant activity which is why it is perfect for weight-loss and anti-cellulite diets. Millet can be a really great breakfast too. You can also mix it with other grains like quinoa or amaranth and add some berries and soya or rice milk. Eating millet for breakfast will give you all the energy you need to start your day.

I also like it with veggies or even in salads. Millet in salads will definitely fill you up and you will not feel like: "hmm had this salad and now feel like hungry again, time to grab some chocolate bar or crisps!"

Azuki

Adzuki beans are high in good carbohydrates and dietary fiber, rich in protein and several vitamins and minerals. Like any other legumes, if combined with integral grain, adzuki beans form a great natural source of protein (perfect for vegetarians). It is a great salad component as well.

More recommendations:

1. Whole grains: rich in fibers, they will prevent food cravings (like the above mentioned quinoa). Great in puddings!

2. Bananas: instead of having a croissant or toast, have a banana. It can be a great quick breakfast if you are on the go. If you are craving for something sweet, try this recipe instead.

54

It's natural, no added sugar, plus it has anti-inflammatory properties:
-Half banana (or 1 small)
-Half cup coconut milk
-Juice of 1 lemon
-1/2 teaspoon maca powder for more energy
-1/2 teaspoon cinnamon and nutmeg
-1 inch fresh ginger

Blend in a blender, stir and enjoy! Sweeten with stevia if you wish.

3. Papaya: it is high in antioxidant beta-carotene, which can help prevent damage to body tissue. It's great in salads and smoothies or even as a quick snack.

4. Pomegranate, lemon and grapefruit juices: cleanse the lymphatic system with super refreshing alkalizing drinks!

5. Ginger: you can spice up all your meals and desserts without having to use table sugar, or table salt that only add to cellulite appearance. It will boost the blood flow and help to cleanse out toxins and make you feel stronger.

6. Berries: boost your skin's collagen levels.

7. Asparagus: circulation-boosting properties that reduce cellulite. Great in stir-fries or with guacamole.

8. Avocadoes: rich in essential fatty acids which can help to strengthen skin and keep it supple and elastic.

9. Oily fish: they reduce inflammation and boost the cardiovascular and lymphatic systems, making them a good choice for keeping cellulite at bay.

10 Fruits: Pineapples reduce water retention and slow digestion, apples burn fat and therefore are good for weight-

loss diets, carrots i m p r o v e general tone of the skin and are good antioxidants Ginger is also a nice ingredient in juices.

More recommendations to kill cellulite:

Yerba Mate

The herb yerba mate contains a group of natural substances called methylxanthines. They are fat burning and are also effective appetite suppressants. Don't overdo it as they are very powerful stimulants as well; if you are caffeine-sensitive, don't use yerba mate. If you have any Argentinean friends, ask them to teach you how to prepare mate. No one else will be able to teach you how to do it the proper way!

Soya Lecithin

Soya lecithin has long been known to improve circulation and energy levels. It brings significant positive changes in peripheral circulation as well. It is both recommended to improve memory and fight stress and speed up all kinds of recoveries. Soya Lecithin is very helpful if you have an active lifestyle, when you need that extra boost of energy. I used to take it before my exams when I was at Uni. Maybe it was placebo effect, but I found it very helpful!.

Ginkgo Biloba

Many experts recommend ginkgo biloba extracts to stimulate microcirculation and I am sure they do a great job when used in correct portions over a certain period of time. As in case of all herbs or natural food supplements, I would suggest you consult your physician first. As for ginkgo biloba, my ophthalmologist, who is also a homeopath and a phytotherapist told me that very often people abuse it and self-medicate with for different purposes. She had had the whole series of patients developing sever eye problems as a result. This is why I always repeat the same line all over again: **natural therapies can never be abused** and just as if in case of standard medications and drugs, they should never be used for self-medication.

Still, I mention it as I know people who were using ginkgo biloboa with great results and improved their microcirculation and other conditions.

Spiruline(Spirulina)

If you have never heard of algas before, I suggest you discover alga called spiruline. You can get either spiruline tablets (normally taken 15- 30 minutes before meals) or get spiruline powder that can be mixed with juices or certain meals, salads, etc.

Spiruline is also used in weight-loss diets and is recommended for people suffering from low energy levels. It is great for active people and if you use it before your workout you will burn more calories. It is not an excessive stimulant like a ginseng plant for example and so even people who are prone to anxiety can take it as it does not increase the heartbeat. Make sure you buy good-quality, organic spiruline and research the brand.

Green Juices

Here, I refer to green, chlorophyll rich juices extracted from leafy greens, vegetables and fruits low in sugar. Remember that juicing fruit rich in sugar is not good for you. It's better to use fruit for smoothies (and drink it with its fiber) or eat it.

Try to juice cucumbers, tomatoes, beets, spinach, kale, fennel and fruits like lemons, limes and grapefruit. These are very alkaline-forming in the body.

If you want to learn more about juicing, specifically for weight loss, and do it the right way, check out the following article on my blog (also available in audio): www.holisticwellnessproject.com/blog/weight-loss/alkaline-juicing-for-weight-loss/

Chapter 7

Exercise

If it is not your regular habit yet, you will need to start working out as soon as possible. Exercise routines should be something enjoyable and something that you really love. For example, I really love outdoor activities and in the summertime I try to be out as much as possible, whereas in the winter I normally catch up with pilates classes and some cardio routine at the gym. I am not really good at water sports but I really love jogging and long walks in the mountains. I hate team sports like volleyball or football but I love cycling! There are so many options out there for different personal preferences. Choose sports that you love and that really make you feel good. Think of the best activity for yourself. Maybe you can enroll in some classes together with a friend? There are also other benefits: going to the gym can help you meet some new people and get some extra inspiration for a really healthy lifestyle. You will also feel more energy and zest for life and will reduce risks of anxiety, insomnia and stress. Not to mention a really fit, sexy body that comes as a main benefit.

Choose your favorite physical activity and burn off cellulite while having fun:

1. Running
2. Swimming
3. Brisk walking
4. Pilates
5. Some energetic variations of yoga
6. Cycling
7. Aerobics
8. Dancing
9. Martial Arts
10. Tennis

Now that you have changed your dietary habits and feel much more energetic and motivated, it is definitely a good time to start exercising. You have already invested time and money in investigating and learning how to eliminate cellulite which is why you can't afford to waste your efforts now and give up on regular exercise routine.

Regular exercise will speed up the process of reducing cellulite and will make an excellent team with natural therapies and healthy foods that were mentioned in this book. Make sure you move your body every day. If you can't workout for an hour, just do 15 minutes. Remember when I mentioned getting off a subway one stop before my final destination so as to at least walk for about 15- 20 minutes? Or maybe, you can commit to a series of squats every morning (I do my squats first thing in the morning, and I stick to it even when I travel, it's so easy- no equipment needed!).

What really motivates me to do exercise is my mind. I know that my mind will reap the main benefit. I will feel MENTALLY STRONGER and I will feel much better about my body as well. I will also have a healthy body and look fit. I can't see myself living in a different way as it has become a part of my lifestyle. However it wasn't always like that. I have struggled with procrastination very often, trust me! I would look for excuses like:

- *Well, I can go to the gym tomorrow*
- *Might just stay at home and chill*
- *I am too tired to work out*
- *I will work out at home later on* (I find it difficult to work out at home, I know myself and I know that it's something I just don't do. I can meditate at home or do yoga but no workouts). But I didn't of course. I would 'chill out' on my sofa with my cute little cats instead (they don't have cellulite!).

I encourage you to change your mind set about exercise. Re-program yourself. Turn pain and effort into pleasure. For now, forget about cellulite. Just do yourself a favor and change your lifestyle. Enjoy every little change that you make. And let me repeat again:

It all starts on a cellular level. Think about it: nothing can actually stop you from taking action and healing every single cell of your body. Get back in balance. Invest in your body and let it work for you.

At the end of this book, you will find some specific anti-cellulite home workouts as well as yoga and pilates exercises that I do and recommend.

Chapter 8

Manual Lymphatic Drainage

I hope that after reading the previous chapter you have already made the decision to get back on this track and become a physically active person in order to kill off cellulite without warning.

Now it's time to get treated with manual lymphatic drainage which is a type of therapy a bit different than a classical or Swedish massage. It especially addresses the problems connected with cellulite, strae, edema, water retention and poor circulation.

I recommend that you find a massage therapist qualified in manual lymphatic drainage, as this technique will speed up the process of cellulite reduction.It is also used as an additional treatment to burn fat and to lose weight and it also alleviates fluid retention. Of course, let me tell you that going only for massage won't do miracles. It is a great, natural addition to the therapies and activities that were already discussed in this book and it can also be a great reward for you. If you can't afford regular massage, you can check out local massage schools, very often they are looking for volunteering patients; all they ask for is your body. Lymphatic Drainage is not like osteopathy or quiropractise so don't worry- you won't get hurt and your bones will stay where they are. Actually, even though it is called " massage", Lymphatic Drainage is not really a massage as there are no real massage movements like kneading for example. The sensation that you feel is as if you had a little cat gently moving its little paws and up and down your body. It's hard to explain in words actually, you should just try it for yourself.

You will also find this massage technique very relaxing as it is extremely soft and slow. There are no oils used in this technique; it is performed on a 'dry' skin. There are many beauty salons using machines that apparently do something similar to lymphatic drainage, but let me tell you one thing: nothing compares to human touch and human dedication.

Manual Lymphatic Drainage is a technique that was first created by a Danish doctor, Emil Vodder around 1933. Originally, he was investigating the lymphatic system to find an effective technique to help his patients who were suffering from chronic colds and sinusitis. Before the Second World War, he was running a clinic in the South of France, where his wife doctor Estrid Vodder specialized in Beauty Medicine.

The Lymphatic Drainage technique that was a result of their investigation and the medical experience was a huge success both in health and beauty treatments. Today, it is used in the whole range of natural beauty procedures as well as for the lymphatic system dysfunctions.

Try to treat yourself to a lymphatic drainage session once a week; it can be a great form of celebrating your new healthy lifestyle and getting a reward for your cellulite burning efforts. Manual lymphatic drainage can definitely speed up the whole process of cellulite elimination and is undoubtedly the easiest and the most enjoyable technique that I mention in this book.

Its multiple benefits are:

1. It activates the natural process of cleansing the bodily tissues and strengthens the immune system

2. It helps fight stress and some nervous system dysfunctions (insomnia, anxiety, and lack of concentration)

3. It is a great natural therapy to fight acne and eczemas (it cleans the subcutaneous tissues)

4. It alleviates sinusitis

5. It helps to get rid of toxins that accumulate in muscles and articulations, and it prevents arthritis

6. It eliminates the sensation of heaviness, being tired; it is indicated in cases of water retention, varicose veins etc.

7. It forms part of natural beauty treatments: facial (wrinkles, eye bags, elasticity loss), and bodily anti-cellulite treatments, skin-invigorating treatments, weight-loss etc.

If you have never tried the Lymphatic Drainage massage, it's time you give yourself a gift and find your local Massage Angel who is trained in this marvelous technique.

You will be amazed at the results!

Of course, this technique is effective if combined with a healthy diet and exercise.
Try to change your lifestyle first and use anti-cellulite treatments like massage and oils to stimulate the process and speed up detoxification that should first be achieved via a balanced nutrition and exercise.

Seek long-term results and kill off cellulite forever! What's the point of repeating the same, boring process again and again and spending a fortune so as to end up where you were before? Trust me, I have been there myself and from my own experience I suggest you choose the long-term success that normally comes as a free bonus or a full packet with a really great product called Holistic Health

Chapter 10: BONUS: Eliminating Cellulite with the Alkaline Diet

As we have stated in the previous chapters, in these changing times, people are eating more and more processed, sugary, and acidic food. This causes them not only to have cellulite, but also to suffer from several disorders, such as obesity, migraines, fatigue, etc. It is sad that many people don't make the connection between diet and disease and opt to take medication, when all it takes is a few dietary changes for them to regain good health.

For instance, one of the causes of cellulite is being overly acidic, and cellulite can be easily reduced with an alkaline-friendly diet.

In this chapter, you will be given a crash course on why over-acidification is bad for your body and how following the alkaline diet (or the alkaline diet inspired) can reverse such effects.

If you are new to this concept, download this free complimentary eBook that also includes recipes and charts:

www.bitly.com/AlkalineMarta

Let's just cover the very basics. There are so many benefits to following the alkaline diet. Yes, you will get rid of your cellulite, but you can also feel more invigorated, your immune system will be stronger, and you will be healthier.

Why is acidity bad?

The natural pH of the fluids in the human body is slightly alkaline. When the fluids are slightly alkaline, most cells function optimally. However, eating a lot of acidic food (including processed cereals, sodas, fast food, coffee, dairy, cakes, meat, sugar, alcohol, chemicals, and preservatives) can speed up the aging process. Aging most easily manifests on the skin through wrinkles, cellulite, etc.

This aging is caused by the body's natural response to over-acidity. Human cells can pull the alkaline calcium and magnesium ions from the bones to neutralize the increased acidity. However, this weakens the integrity of the bones and may cause osteoporosis. Iodine is also taken from soft tissues, which could lead to weight gain and diabetes.

Obesity and being overweight are also the effects of over-acidification. Acids can really harm vital organs, such as the heart and lungs; therefore, your body produces fat cells to carry these harmful acids away from your vital organs. Fat actually saves your life.

On the other hand, an overly-acidic body could be a welcome home to several types of yeast and fungi. These microbes will feed on your nutrients, leaving you excessively thin and disease-prone. We don't want that situation either, do we?

Are acid foods always acid in taste?

Nope. For example, some citrus fruits like lemons and limes, are acidic by taste, but provide an alkalizing effect on your body. Why? It's simple- they are rich in alkaline minerals and low in sugar. On the other hand, avocados do not taste acidic, but they create an alkaline environment inside your body once digested. To sum- we do not care about the alkalinity or acidity of foods before they enter our body. We need to know what effect they have on your body once digested.

What's good about eating more alkaline?

Having an alkaline diet will stabilize your body chemistry. This means that you will be neither overweight nor underweight, since your body will regain its natural ability to maintain its own weight.

The alkaline diet may also help people suffering from allergies. Since allergies are often a symptom of a malfunctioning digestive system, many types of amino acids are just floating about inside your body, which aggravates the condition. Alkalizing is one way to help balance the environment in your body, thereby preventing hypersensitivity.

What food can you eat to reverse acidity or maintain alkalinity?

Your body has its own system (called "buffers") which naturally maintains the pH at a certain range. Eating more alkaline (and drinking more alkaline) , however, will prevent your body from needing to do the regulation. Instead, the body can focus on other things, such as digestion and providing energy.

It's a good thing that acidity can be easily reversed by choosing your food wisely. The alkaline diet advocates the consumption of raw vegetables, some fruits (especially lemons, limes, tomatoes, avocados, and grapefruits), and natural, unprocessed, gluten-free grains like quinoa as well as clean, unprocessed foods in general. The best "alkalizer" is lemon, which you should drink as juice in warm water at the start of the day. Lemons are able to flush away the harmful byproducts of the liver. To prevent tooth enamel damage, use a straw.

Again, if you are new to the alkaline diet, and wish to find out which foods are alkaline/acid forming, please download the charts at:

www.bitly.com/AlkalineMarta

Get my charts, print them out and stick to your fridge.

Furthermore, greens are a great way to balance an acidic meal (for example meat). Try mixing spinach, lettuce, celery, parsley, kale, fresh ginger, and lemon in a juice to boost your alkalinity.

This is how your plate should look:

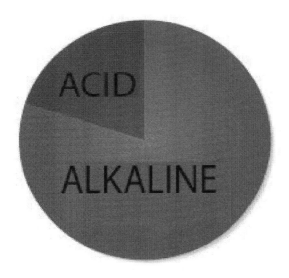

Additionally, almonds and carrots are highly recommended as healthy food choices and snacks. Both of these are high in Vitamin A and antioxidants, which are great for your eyesight, skin, and teeth. Since both of them have a low glycemic index, your insulin levels won't spike. (Studies have shown that consistently having high insulin levels leads to cellulite formation.)

Please note that although having the alkaline diet is good for you, it's not about eating 100% alkaline (uff, this makes it a bit easier, right? You don't need to be perfect). Most health professionals and alkaline diet gurus, like for example Doctor Robert O.Young, recommend striking a 75-80% alkaline and 20-25% acid balance in your diet. Of course, not everyone is the same, but that is the general idea. People with severe health problems may be advised to eat more alkaline (more than 80%) or do a specific alkaline detox, but this is not a topic of this book.

Back to our enemy...
We already know that cellulite refers to the deposition of fat in certain parts of the body that causes the skin above it to pucker out.

There are actually 4 grades of cellulites:
- Grade 1: Cellulite is not visible, even when the skin is pinched.
- Grade 2: Cellulite is not visible when sitting or standing. However, an "orange peel" texture is observable when the skin is pinched.
- Grade 3: Cellulite is visible when standing up but could disappear when lying down.
- Grade 4: Cellulite is visible when standing and when lying down.

There are many factors that lead to cellulite formation. These include:
- Genes
- Eating nutritionally poor food
- Eating unhealthy food
- Sedentary lifestyle
- Slow metabolism
- Fad dieting
- Dehydration
- A high amount of body fat
- Hormone imbalances
- Thickness of skin
- Poor circulation

Can acidification cause cellulite?

As mentioned previously, fat deposits can occur when the body is overly acidic. Sticking to the alkaline diet can reduce the formation of such fat deposits. Moreover, the alkaline diet could also help in solving hormone imbalances, such as in the case of fat-forming insulin.

How can eating eradicate cellulite?

The idea behind any kind of diet is eating the *right* types of food. Try out a plant-based diet with lots of veggies, fruits, and alkaline grains. These foods include: high protein quinoa, millet, amaranth, high fiber foods, nuts (almonds, walnuts), Omega 3-rich foods (flax, chia), and (if you are not a vegetarian) good quality organic meats and fish (occasionally) like grass fed meat, free range chicken. These help in bringing your body back to balance and in eradicating cellulite. Acid foods (like meat and fish) should not be more than 20- max 30% of your diet.

Fresh fruits and vegetables are great in boosting circulation. Since the blood flow is good, blood can reach even the smaller vessels near the skin cells. The blood can then feed your skin with the proper nutrients and remove the buildup of toxins which may cause cellulite.

Alkaline citrus fruits like lemons, limes and grapefruits, contain high levels of vitamin C and bioflavonoids which aid in improving the flow of blood and in strengthening the walls of the capillaries. Watermelons and tomatoes are rich in lycopene, which prevents the build-up of plaque – the substance which hinders blood flow to the arteries. Pumpkin seeds have Vitamin E, which also aids in circulation. Nuts contain niacin, which is proven to prevent circulation problems. Garlic also prevents plaque formation.

If you want to follow the alkaline diet, remember to add as many alkaline vegetables (also juiced or blended) and alkaline fruits. These are lemons, limes, tomatoes, avocados, pomegranates, coconut and grapefruits, the rest of fruits is moderately acidic, but of course, you should still have them. As mentioned in the previous chapters, they are full of vital nutrients.

What are other ways of preventing cellulite?

Aside from having a good diet, you should also ensure that you engage in regular, daily exercise- it is also a part of the alkaline lifestyle. Yes, when you you're your body (especially outdoors activities), you also alkalize your body and mind. Exercising for at least 15 minutes a day is better than exercising for 2 hours on the weekends. Exercising promotes the circulation of blood throughout the entire body. Since cellulite can be the effect of poor circulation (cellulite tends to form in areas with the least circulation), exercising can prevent its formation. Exercising doesn't even need to be hard. Simply brisk walking, running, or swimming is enough to remind your blood to keep moving around.

Cut down on refined and processed food. Also, try to avoid sweeteners, additives, dairy and high fat products, and sugars.

If you have a desk job, be sure to take occasional breaks and walk and talk with people rather than scroll through your Facebook feed or watching videos (not judging, I have been guilty of it as well).

Don't diet too much or too hard. Health professionals sometimes say that "less is more," especially for the ladies. Be good on yourself. Instead of trying to be 100% perfect, aim to be 70% awesome and 30% relaxed. This will allow some space for occasional treats without "guilt-trips "and stress.

Alkaline Recipes

Try out a few of these alkaline recipes to get rid of cellulite.

Tossed Salad in Olive Oil

Ingredients
- 2 tbsp olive oil
- 1/3 cup tahini
- 1-2 cloves of garlic
- ½ lemon – get the juice
- Salt (to taste)
- 3 tbsp parsley
- Water
- 6 tomatoes
- 1 cucumber

Steps
1. Mix the first 6 ingredients in a salad bowl.
2. Add enough water to thin the tahini.
3. Make into a dressing by stirring thoroughly.
4. Take the cucumber and tomatoes. Dice.
5. Add diced cucumber and tomatoes into the mixture.
6. Toss.
7. Sit for an hour.
8. Enjoy!

Fresh Almond Milk

Ingredients
- 1 bowl water
- 4 cups raw almonds

Materials
- Cheese cloth (to strain the milk)

Steps
1. Soak the almonds in a bowl of water overnight.
2. In the morning, drain the almonds using a strainer.
3. Fill your blender to 1/3 full (around 2 cups) of the almonds.
4. Add pure water until your blender is filled.
5. Fit a cheese cloth over the mouth of a bowl or pan.
6. Drain the blended almonds.
7. Squeeze the almond mush with your hands to get as much milk through the cloth or strain as you can (the almond mush itself can also be used as a wonderful body scrub).
8. Thin with enough water to achieve your desired consistency.
9. Store in the refrigerator. This can last for up to 3 days.

Grassoup

Ingredients
- 2-3 English cucumbers – get the juice
- 1-2 cups of fresh almond milk or coconut milk
- 1-2 young Thai coconuts – get the water by opening the fruit and draining the water. You might want to eat the meat later on.
- 1 tbsp fresh dill – cut into small strips
- Dehydrated red bell pepper powder (optional)

Steps
1. Prepare the dehydrated red bell pepper powder:
2. Place slices of red bell pepper (around ¼" thick) in a dehydrator.
3. Dry until you can snap them crisply. This usually takes around 24 hours.
4. Place in a blender. Grind until they're a fine powder.
5. Store in an airtight container.
6. Combine all ingredients.
7. Consume immediately.
8. Don't be afraid to experiment.
9. For a creamier soup, add more almond milk.
10. For less sweet soup, lessen the coconut water and red bell pepper powder.

Almost Alkaline Smoothie (Sweet Treat!)

Ingredients
- 1 cup coconut water
- 2 tbsp hemp seeds
- 1 handful baby spinach
- 1 tbsp ground flax seeds
- ½ banana
- 1 tbsp. ground chia seeds
- ½ apple
- 1 handful berries (blackberries, blueberries, strawberries – your choice!)
- ½ lemon – get the juice

Steps
1. Mix all ingredients in a blender.
2. Blend until smooth.
3. Drink immediately.

Lime Shake

Ingredients
- ½ avocado
- 1 cucumber
- 1-2 handfuls of baby spinach
- 8-12 ice cubes
- 3-4 peeled limes
- Raw green stevia (adjust according to taste)

Steps
1. Combine all ingredients in a blender.
2. Set the blender on high.
3. Blend until smooth.
4. Drink immediately.

Ginger and Lemon Tea

Ingredients
- 2 cups of water
- ½ lemon – get the juice
- Ginger, grated (optional)

Steps
1. Heat up the water until warm.
2. Add the lemon juice.
3. (optional) Garnish with ginger.
4. Enjoy while hot!

Note: Ginger can really warm up your body. You may opt to skip it, especially during hot, summer months.

There you have it. With all those recipes and with your newfound knowledge in all things alkaline, you finally have the power to eliminate cellulite – safely and naturally!

Chapter10: BONUS: Eliminate Cellulite with Yoga, Pilates and Physical Activity

Yoga can significantly improve your physical health by improving muscle tone and decreasing the fat that contributes to the formation of cellulite.

For instance, you can do lunging poses while standing to strengthen your thigh muscles and buttocks. You can also do twisting poses to aid in your digestion and waste elimination as well as stimulate your internal organs.

You can do inverted poses to strengthen your circulatory system and improve fluid drainage. In addition, your enhanced breathing can improve nutrient and oxygen circulation in your body.

When you practice yoga, your lymph can move more freely through your fatty areas; thus, flushing away toxins and reduce cellulite. So if you want to reduce your cellulite, do the following yoga poses on a regular basis. Do not forget to warm up before exercising and cool down afterwards.

Supported Shoulder Stand

To do this pose, lie down on a mat while resting your shoulders on a folded blanket. Your head should be one to two inches lower than your shoulders. Push your palms against the mat and bend your knees. Lift your feet, lower back, and buttocks off the matt and bring your legs upwards. Then, bend your elbows and put your palms against your lower back as you lift your legs and bring your feet towards the ceiling. Hold this position for thirty seconds and work up to five minutes.

Half Shoulder Stand

To do this pose, lie down and let your arms rest alongside your torso. Next, bend your knees and curl them up towards your forehead. Put your hands beneath your hips for support. Keep your elbows on the ground and stay in this position for eight to ten breaths. Finally, release your knees slowly and gently roll your back down to the ground.

Standing Forward Bend

Stand with feet apart and bend forward, hinging at your hips. Keep your knees slightly bent while you place your chest on your upper thighs and your head towards the ground. Then, engage your quadriceps muscles and straighten your legs slowly. See to it that your knees do not lock and your hips remain over the center of your feet. Hold this position for five to eight slow and deep breaths.

Plow Pose

To do this pose, do the Half Shoulder Stand first. Straighten your legs and extend them backwards. Your toes should rest on the floor. Then, straighten your arms and reach for the floor with your palms facing downwards. Hold this position for eight to ten breaths. Finally, bring your knees to your original position and gently roll your back down to the ground.

Eagle Pose

Slightly bend your knees to cross your right leg over your left leg. If possible, double cross it behind your left ankle or calf. Then, place your right arm under your left arm and put your hands together. Squeeze your thighs tightly as you pull your belly towards your spine. Sink down lower and slightly bend at your knee. Hold this position for five breaths and repeat with your legs and arms reversed.

Chair Pose

Stand with feet together and toes touching. Keep your ankles a bit apart and bend at your knees. Pull your hips backwards as if sitting on a chair and lift your chest upwards. While doing this, lift your arms upwards and lengthen them through your fingertips. Keep your shoulders relaxed and hold your abdominal muscles in. Sit as far back as you can and aim to make a ninety-degree angle with your legs. Hold this position for five to eight breaths before you stand up. Repeat.

Bridge Pose

Lie down. Keep your knees bent and feet on the ground. Relax your glutes, tuck your tailbone, and lift your hips upwards. To reach a wider stretch, you can push your shoulders underneath and interlock your hands beneath your hips. Press your fists onto the ground, tighten your hamstring, core muscles, and buttocks. Hold this position for five to eight breaths and slowly lower to the ground. Repeat two more times.

Cow Face Pose

Begin by dropping down on your knees and hands and sliding your right leg backwards to cross over your left leg. Then, squeeze at your inner thighs and open your feet. Sit between your heels until you feel a release around your buttocks and hip region. Also feel a stretch around your thighs. Hold this position for as many seconds as you want, although eight to ten breaths are better. Repeat the process with your other leg.

Downward-Facing Dog

Bend forward into a forward fold and put your hands on the ground. Step backwards and raise your hips. It is alright if you cannot keep your feet on the ground. Try to pedal your feet and come onto your toes so you can settle into the stretch.

Warrior I

To do this pose, start with the Downward Facing Dog pose. Put a foot forward until it is perpendicular with your other foot. Rise up and bring your hips forward. Raise your hands upward while you stay careful that your front knees do not go over your toes. Keep your back leg straight and repeat the process on the other side.

Warrior II

Stand with your feet together, and then lift your left leg behind you. Tip your weight forward onto your right leg. Lift your left leg while you drop your torso and head so your body and left leg is perpendicular to your right leg and parallel to the ground. Keep your hands at your sides and ensure that your left hip, toes, and thigh remain facing downwards. Keep your right kneecap lifted. Hold this position for five breaths before you switch legs and repeat the process.

Seated Forward Fold

Sit down with your feet at the front. Make sure that your feet stay fixed at that position. Then, bend forward from your hips and maintain a straight back. If possible, try to reach for your toes. Otherwise, you can simply use a strap or towel to further your stretch.

Seated Twist

Sit up straight and cross your knees. Inhale as you lift your hands upwards, and exhale as you bring your left hand behind you and your right hand towards your left knee. Gaze over your shoulder and breathe deeper. Repeat the process on the other side.

Pilates to Reduce Cellulite

Pilates was developed by Joseph Pilates in the late twentieth century and was extremely popular in the United States. It improves flexibility, develops endurance and control, and builds strength. It puts emphasis on breathing, alignment, and improving balance and coordination. Its system allows the modification of a variety of exercises from beginner to advanced levels.

Performing Pilates is another way to reduce your cellulite. In fact, the American Council on Exercise suggests doing two to three sessions per week. Pilates is also advisable for those who do not have cellulite as it can dramatically reduce their likelihood of having it.

This exercise is truly a great way to work all your muscles along with your core. You can use a Pilates reformer, which is a custom contraption that features pulleys and springs to add resistance and facilitate movement, or work on a mat and simply rely on your body weight for resistance.

How to Do Pilates

Start by performing five pelvic lifts to target your buttocks muscles. Lie down on your back, bend your knees, and bring your arms at your sides. Breathe out as you slowly raise your buttocks and squeeze your glutes. Then, breathe in and lower your back slowly. You can repeat this movement with a few variations. As you come up, you can hold the position for five breaths. Focus on releasing and contracting your buttocks. Lower your body down to the ground and repeat the process for five more times.

In order to reduce the cellulite on your outer thighs, work your abductors. Lie down on your left side and bend your knees to ninety degrees. Keep your ankles together and move your right knee away from your left leg. Close and open it for ten repetitions. Then, lift both your right ankle and knee to work your outer thigh muscles more deeply. Do ten repetitions and repeat the same moves on your right side. Do these exercises two to three times per week.

If you want to know more about mat exercises or how to use the reformer, enroll yourself in a Pilates class. The fees for Pilates classes generally depend on the degree of attention that you receive and your usage of equipment. Classes that offer mat exercises alone typically cost less than classes that involve using the reformer. You may get a discount if you enroll in a studio that offers multiple sessions.

Here are some Pilates exercises you can try to reduce your cellulite:

The 100's

Warming up before exercising is crucial to avoid broken bones or injuries. The 100's is a great Pilates warm up because it allows your blood to flow freely as well as warms up your core. It is beneficial for your core, hips, thighs, arms, and buttocks. To do this exercise, lie down and press your spine on your mat. Then, lift up your legs and come to a tabletop pose.

Keep your lower abdomen engaged and stretch your arms. Lift your neck and head up and look at your navel. Bring your legs to a forty-five degree angle position and pump your arms up and down. Inhale for five counts and exhale for another five counts. Repeat this exercise for ten times until you have pumped your arms one hundred times.

Leg Circle and Serving Tray

To do this exercise, lower your neck and head to your mat. Extend one leg upwards and the other downwards. Flex your right foot while you bring extend your left leg outwards. Visualize yourself having a serving tray over your legs. Then, bend down your right knee and imagine balancing the tray. Engage your buttocks and inner thighs. Finally, pull your belly button inwards and steady your hips. Repeat this exercise for eight to ten sets.

To do the leg circle, point the toes of your right foot upwards and circle your leg in a clockwise direction five times. Likewise, circle it in a counter-clockwise direction five times. Do not let your torso and hips move while you do this. Do the same thing with your left leg. Leg circle exercises are beneficial for your buttocks, hips, abdomen, calves, outer thighs, and inner thighs.

Climb a Tree

To do this exercise, you have to bring your leg backwards and keep your abdominal muscles engaged. Position yourself in a way as if you are trying to climb a tree. Make sure that your shoulders remain soft. Use your core muscles and not your arm muscles to climb upwards. Once you are in a sitting position, curl beneath your tailbone and tuck in your lower abdomen, and then lower yourself slowly back to the ground. Do this exercise for five more times before switching to your other leg. Climb a Tree is perfect for your scapula, thighs, and lower abdomen.

Single Leg Stretch

To do this exercise, lie on a mat and lift your neck and head upwards. Then, bring your right knee towards your chest and bring your left leg to a forty-five degree position. Do the same thing with your other leg. Continue switching legs for eight repetitions. This Pilates workout is great for your hips, arms, buttocks, thighs, and abdomen.

Double Leg Stretch

To do this exercise, bring your knees towards your chest and lift your neck and head upwards as you inhale. Then, extend your legs and arms away from your body while you exhale. Bring your arms to your sides while you bring your legs towards your chest. Do this for eight repetitions and never allow your head to drop as you extend your arms. Engage your abdomen and press your back against your mat. This Pilates exercise is great for your arms, thighs, hips, and abdomen.

Other Workouts to Reduce Cellulite

You can also reduce your cellulite by walking and weight lifting. Regular brisk walking is actually a great way to tone your thighs and improve your overall well-being. When walking, decide on which routes you are going to take. You have to map out a selection of one and a half, two and a half, and three-mile courses.

You can walk or drive around your chosen route to measure its distance. If you want to reap additional benefits, include inclines and hills in your workout. See to it that you set aside at least forty-five minutes per day for your walk, but do not forget to have a rest day.

Of course, you need to wear the right clothes for your workouts, and wear good quality running or walking shoes. Make sure that you also walk at a pace that is comfortable for you. If you are a newbie, do not push yourself too hard. If you believe you are up for advanced exercises, you can include jogging in your routine.

Do not forget to warm up and cool down before and after exercising to avoid injury. Keep in mind that posture is also crucial. You have to keep your chin held high and your shoulders back. Look straight ahead and walk in a natural manner. Quicken your pace and allow your arms to swing.

If you find yourself short of breath or your legs start to become stiffer while you walk, slow down a little. If you start to feel dizzy, stop and regain your equilibrium.

Aside from walking, lifting weights can also help you reduce your cellulite. A workout routine that involves weights can actually improve your overall effort to eliminate cellulite. When you build muscle, you are able to burn calories quickly and achieve weight loss. This improves the condition of your skin.

If you incorporate free weights, resistance bands, and weight machines into your weight training, you will be able to build more muscle and boost your metabolic rate. Having a fast metabolism is great because it causes your body to burn lots of calories as well as tap into its stored fat supply.

With resistance training, you can remodel your skin tissue and smooth out your cellulite. Also, losing weight can relieve the pressure between fat and its connective tissue; thus, reducing the presence of cellulite.

If you want to improve your muscle tone and burn excess fat, exercise with weights twenty to forty-five minutes three to five times per week. Also walk forty-five minutes daily three times per week at a pace that can increase your pulse at fifty to sixty percent.

Home Workouts – Squats and Lunges

If you cannot go to the gym because you have a hectic schedule, the nearest gym is still too far from your home, or you do not want to endure a stressful commute, do not worry because you can simply exercise at home.

Squats and lunges are basic exercises that reduce cellulite, and the best thing about them is that you can do them without using any weights or any kind of equipment whatsoever. You can use your body weight, however you can use weights to increase the difficulty later. A word of caution before you proceed though, you have to ensure that you do not put too much stress on your knees or lower back so you will not get any injuries that will sideline you for a long time.

To perform a squat, stand up with your back straight and bend your knees. Your thighs should stay parallel to the ground. Push your glutes backwards as if you are trying to sit on a chair. And then, use your leg muscles to come back up slowly to a standing position.

It is ideal that you perform three sets of twenty to forty squats three times per week. You can also use barbells or dumbbells to add intensity and make your workouts more challenging.

Squats work your leg muscles, including your hamstrings, lower leg muscles, and quadriceps. They also work your gluteus maximus, rectus abdominus, and erector spinae muscles. Likewise, lunges are great for tightening your legs and buttocks. You can try the following lunges:

Walking Lunge with Bicep Curl

To perform this exercise, stand up straight with your feet together while holding two five to ten-pound dumbbells at your sides. Bring your left leg forward and curl your dumbbells towards your shoulders. Remember to keep your elbows as close to your body as much as possible.

Then, lower your hips towards the floor and bend both of your knees to about ninety degrees. Keep your back knee close to but not actually touching the ground. Also, try to keep your front knee directly over your ankle. Your back knee should point towards the ground.

Push off using your right foot and move forward to your starting position. Lower your dumbbells to your side to complete one repetition. Finally, step forward and repeat the process with your right leg. Complete two to three sets of fifteen repetitions to have a good workout.

Revenge Lunge

This exercise targets your quads and glutes. To begin, stand with your feet apart and arms at your sides. Hold your dumbbells at your sides. Then, lunge backwards with your right foot and bend both of your knees at ninety degrees. Hold this position for one second and go back to start. Repeat the process and do twelve to fifteen repetitions.

What to do when you don't feel motivated to work out:

- Be sure to have a fitness vision board with images that inspire you to take action.

- Trick your brain: instead of procrastinating about a 1 hour workout, tell your mind: hey, it's easy. I will commit myself to a simple 5 minute workout and I will do it now. 5 minutes is better than nothing and it will make you feel good and more motivated. I do this trick very often, and most of the time I end up working out for more than 5 minutes.

- Music: create your favorite playlists, something with an energetic beat to keep you going. If you really can't motivate yourself just start jumping around while shouting out some positive affirmations (sounds weird but it works.)

The best part about home workouts? They are free.
So get started today. Begin with simple squats and go from there.

Conclusion

Thank you again for taking interest in my work.

I hope that I was able to help you find some new holistic ways to eliminate cellulite so as to have the body you have always wanted. I also hope that you managed to change your attitude a bit and made the decision to live a mindful and healthy lifestyle.

Of course, reading this book alone will not be the ultimate cellulite solution: it is necessary to persistently and regularly apply all of the techniques mentioned here. The reward that you will get for your efforts is successfully winning the battle against cellulite in a natural and inexpensive way.

Start applying the techniques as described and make them your everyday routine. The results will be visible sooner than you expect. It feels really good to eat healthy, think healthy and be healthy. I also hope that my book inspired you to take care of yourself in a truly holistic way. If you feel that my book can help your family or friends or you simply enjoyed reading it, please share it.

Finally, if you enjoyed this book, it would be greatly appreciated if you left a review so others can receive the same benefits you have. Your review can help other people take this important step to take care of their health and inspire them to start a new chapter in their lives. At the same time, you can help me serve you and all my other readers even more.

I'd be thrilled to hear from you. I would love to know your top 3 tips! Or at least your chapter or section. As long as I know what you like, I can create more books that will help you on your journey.
Simply visit the link below and write a short review to share your experience. I know you are busy and I would like to thank

you in advance for considering taking a couple of minutes to review this book. Even 1 sentence will do.

Amazon US: www.amazon.com/dp/B00EPOJ5Z8
Amazon UK: www.amazon.co.uk/dp/B00EPOJ5Z8
Amazon CA: www.amazon.ca/dp/B00EPOJ5Z8
Amazon AU: www.amazon.com.au/dp/B00EPOJ5Z8

Or, go to your Amazon orders (digital orders if you read it as a kindle book) and click on my book. Alternatively, you can type: "Marta Tuchowska" in Amazon search bar.
BIG THANKS!

For more information and free holistic resources (motivation, alkaline diet, holistic health, weight loss, aromatherapy, spa, mindfulness, lifestyle and personal development) including podcasts, articles, eBooks and audiobooks, visit:

www.HolisticWellnessProject.com

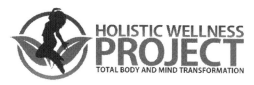

ADDITIONAL RESOURCES FOR ALKALINE WELLNESS MOTIVATION

Looking for more recipes and wellness?

Follow me on Instagram and discover my holistic lifestyle secrets + dozens of alkaline recipes, picks and motivational videos that will help you keep on track throughout the day:

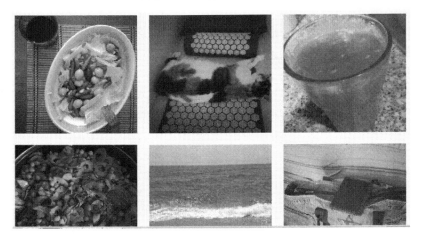

www.instagram.com/Marta_Wellness

More Wellness Books from Marta Tuchowska

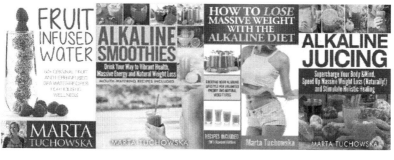

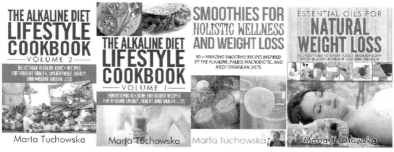

Available in Kindle and Paperback

You will find much, much more at:

www.bitly.com/MartaBooks

www.amazon.com/author/mtuchowska

FINALLY- LET'S KEEP IN TOUCH:

www.instagram.com/Marta_Wellness

www.facebook.com/HolisticWellnessProject

www.twitter.com/Marta_Wellness

www.pinterest.com/martaWellness/

www.udemy.com/u/martatuchowska

www.plus.google.com/+MartaTuchowska

NEED MORE MOTIVATION?

Listen to my podcast:

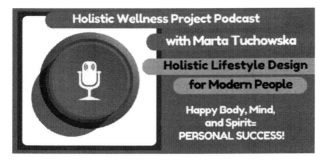

www.holisticwellnessproject.com/blog/podcast

www.holisticwellnessproject.com/blog/alkaline-diet

->most of my articles are **also available in MP3** so that you can feed your mind with positive information even if you are busy.

I wish you wellness, health, and success in whatever it is that you want to accomplish.

With lots of LOVE and positive energy,

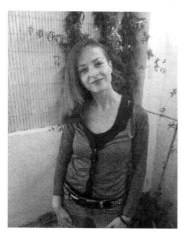

Marta Tuchowska

Founder and CEO of Holistic Wellness Project LTD, Wellness & Lifestyle Coach, Motivational Coach, International Author, Alkaline Diet Advocate, Creator of AlkalineDietLifestyle.com

Certified in Holistic Nutrition, Massage Therapy, Aromatherapy, Reiki II Therapist. Currently studying hypnosis and NLP.

Made in the USA
Lexington, KY
13 March 2016